MIND BODY SECRETS

eBook ISBN: 978-1-958405-80-2
Paperback ISBN: 978-1-958405-79-6
Hardcover ISBN: 978-1-958405-85-7
Library of Congress Control Number: 2023910636
Printed in the United States of America

Interior Design: Marigold2k
Cover Artistry: Amanda Wolf - www.amandawolfcreates.com
Bio Headshot: Jonathan Henniger - www.jonathanhenniger.com
Cover Headshot - Kris Kinsley Hancock - www.nantucketpix.com
Editing: Write2Unite
Published By: Spotlight Publishing House
https://spotlightpublishinghouse.com

Disclaimer: The advice offered in this book is evidence-based science combined with the humanity-based experience we all share. This is not a prescription for your own unique needs in health care. None the less, regardless of your unique situation, learning and adjusting your habits and lifestyle to support your body's needs will reward you in ways you cannot imagine until you go through this journey. This book will help you and your doctors be happier about being with each other. As a doctor and a patient, I offer this gift to patients and doctors alike so we may heal from the broken medical system we unfortunately share. My intention is to help, bring healing, and hope for developing new systems that empower each of us in our unique service spaces, and expand the health potential of mankind for future generations.

www.beatrizolson.com

Endorsements

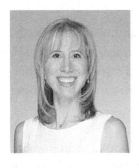

Beatriz Olson, MD has written a book that is heartfelt, empathic, and inspirational — a book informed by her extensive personal and professional experiences that gives the reader a roadmap with guidance, tools, and knowledge to transform one's life — mind, body, and spirit. Reading it has already given me new insights and perspectives to enrich my life.

I highly recommend this excellent book for anyone desiring to live a life of fulfillment and joy.

—Jill R. Baron MD
Integrative and Functional Medicine physician and author of *Don't Mess with Stress*

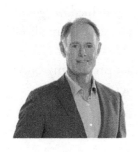

Our highly refined genome, a gift from all who have come before us, provides our bodies with an incredibly resilient physiology. But this is ancestral biology, optimized for the environment of our forebears. And it is the mismatch between our evolution and our current environment that is central to so many of the diseases of our modern world. In *Mind Body Secrets,* Dr. Olson provides the reader the evidence-based tools for revitalization of body, mind and spirit and reconnection to the life enhancing and health sustaining messaging that is our gift from all who have come before.

—David Perlmutter, MD
#1 *New York Times* bestselling author *Grain Brain*

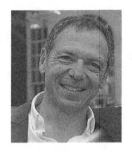

There are many books about how to heal the body, many about how best to eat and many about the advantages of a strong spiritual life. But there is only one I have seen, that combines the knowledge of all three areas, it's this one.

With simple, compelling and insightful words, Dr. Beatriz Olson not only illustrates the incredible advantages of mind, spirit and the body working together, she also shows you in very practical ways how you can start by doing this right now.

Mind Body Secrets is a wonderfully uplifting book, written with passion and compassion for the author herself, who uses her own example (and those of many of her patients) to illustrate what she means by each step she proposes.

—Pedro Simko
Former Head of Western Europe, Publicis Communications and author of *Happy at Work* and *The River*

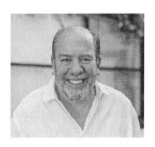

Mind Body Secrets not only helped me get to know my body, but it also showed me how to listen to my body, understand my body and heal my body. In that process my body became my sacred partner in life.

Thank you for this gift, Dr. Beatriz!

—Philip Nicholas,
Chief Creative Officer for Choice Point
Master Coach for the Stress Reset.

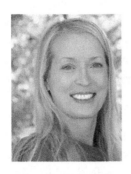

Mind Body Secrets is a must read for every woman interested in improving her health, happiness, and overall wellbeing. Dr. Olson's inspiring personal story is expertly interwoven with her years of medical experience and expertise. As she shares her insight and knowledge of mind-body-medicine you will be taken on an empowering transformational journey.

—Joann Burnham
Founder and Director Dharma Yoga Nantucket, Founder Nantucket Yoga Festival

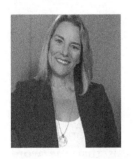

Do you ever wish that your doctor had more experience with fully integrated health strategies of mind-body medicine? And even more so, that they have time to discuss them with you? Dr. Beatriz Olson has spent over three decades studying the secrets of mind-body medicine and wellness and has written this book to share them with you! Reading this book will give your insight and understanding as well as help you get the most out of your visits with your own health care providers."

—Donnica L. Moore MD
President Sapphire Women's Health Group & Editor-in-Chief, Women's Health for Life

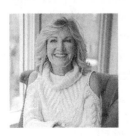

In her book, Beatriz Olson, M.D., has gifted us with the brilliance of over 40 years of medical practice and the humanity and inspiration of her entire life. *Mind Body Secrets* is one of the most comprehensive books available on the wellness of the mind, body, and spirit. Dr. Olson provides the integrative and holistic steps that can help all of us forge sustainable and lasting transformation. Who knew how much our ancestral wiring plays a role in our efforts to deal with excess weight, stress, and relationship challenges? Who knew what we might learn in a psychologist's office or at a spiritual retreat could be expanded on and incorporated into our daily efforts to enhance our vitality? Dr. Olson brings various modalities of healing together into this one priceless book that contains realistic approaches to our wellness, not gimmicks or empty promises. Dr. Olson connects with her readers as she does with her own patients. She is vulnerable and shares her personal stories, making her accessible and relatable. She is a connector, not an aloof knower. She is compassionate and caring and the kind of inspirational example that sets a higher bar for the entire field of medicine. I'm recommending this gem of a book to everyone I know.

—Kim Douglas
Educator, Writer & Editor,
Founder & CEO, Write2Unite

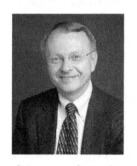

"Knowledge is power." This concept permeates Dr. Olson's book, *Mind Body Secrets*, and a search of the book reveals that the word "knowledge" appears 25 times. Knowing Dr. Olson as I do, this is not surprising.

As an accomplished scientist, researcher and endocrinologist, she has always demanded that our clinical recommendations to our patients are consistent with the best available knowledge, even when they are not yet fully evidence-based. In this book, Dr. Olson explains how knowledge about the evolutionary origins of our physiology and behavior can help us understand how this has become counter-productive in our current environment. By explaining complex body physiology in terms that are understandable to everyone, regardless of their scientific background, this empowers everyone to use this knowledge to understand what drives us to do things that adversely affect our health, and longevity. But knowledge alone is not sufficient to enable us to change our trajectory to a healthier life.

Thorough compelling clinical examples and practical recommendations, Dr. Olson provides blueprints that everyone can follow to improve their lives, but equally importantly to me, the happiness of their lives, by asking critical introspective questions about why we continue to pursue unhealthy lifestyle habits. The critically important message of this book is that if we understand the physiological evolutionary knowledge underlying the unconscientious decisions we all make every day, then we can be empowered to change what we do in response to these drives in order to lead healthier, longer lives.

—Joseph Verbalis MD,
Professor of Medicine
Chief, Endocrinology and Metabolism at Georgetown University
Georgetown-Howard Universities Center for Clinical and Translational Science Washington, DC

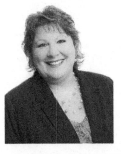

Bravo Dr. Beatriz Olson! You created an informative and practical guide to transform our ancestral Mind and Body to optimal 21st century wellness.

You scientifically validate the nuances of how our bodies are designed to benefit from a holistic care approach. Your melding of science and spirituality will captivate and catapult readers.

—Rev. Maggie Mongan,
CEO Brilliant Breakthroughs, Inc.
Creator of #1 Bestselling Book Series:
Brilliant Breakthroughs for the Small Business Owner

MIND BODY SECRETS

A Medical Doctor's Spiritual and Scientific Guide to Wellness

Dr. Beatriz Olson

SPOTLIGHT
PUBLISHING HOUSE

Goodyear, AZ

To my entelechy,

my matriarchal line,

our daughters,

and future generations.

Contents

Part I. Care of The Mind

Part II. Care of The Body

Part III. Care of The Soul

List of Figures

Foreword

I am delighted to introduce you to *Mind Body Secrets*, Dr. Beatriz Olson's remarkable book on optimal wellness. As the founder of The Institute for Woman-Centered Coaching, Training & Leadership, I have had the privilege of working with countless women on their journeys toward self-discovery and empowerment and can honestly say the issues Dr. Olson addresses in this book affect each and every one of us.

Having had the privilege of witnessing Dr. Olson's visionary leadership, energy and remarkable insights firsthand in our programs and community for many years, I can attest to her experience, expertise, and the authenticity of her calling. Her dedication to sharing her understanding of the root cause of our world's current health crisis with as many people as possible is palpable.

In her 40-year career as a highly regarded integrative medical practitioner and an expert in endocrinology, she has helped thousands of individual patients to overcome illness and disease, excess weight, and the various stresses of our contemporary world. Her extensive research, combined with the wisdom gleaned from Jungian psychotherapy, Buddhist philosophy, and meditation practice, creates a powerful synthesis of knowledge and insight.

In the pages of this book, you will embark on a transformative journey—one that resonates deeply with our shared experiences of living in our fast-paced, rapidly changing world. She sees that we are disconnected from the needs of our bodies, living in our heads, absorbing the relentless persuasive messaging and information bombarding us to do, achieve, and have more. Thus, we no longer feel we can take care of ourselves, and this lack of self-care leads to sickness and distress at multiple levels of our being.

Her book is unique, as it provides a remarkable blueprint for lifelong health that honors the essential interactions between mind, body and spirit founded on evidence-based science, with complimentary medicine approaches, mindfulness, and spirituality, her stories and those of her patients, all held and informed by woman-centered transformation skills.

Dr. Olson's timeless manual has the potential to ignite a quiet revolution for millions—one which supports and enhances Feminine Power principles, enabling women and people everywhere to reclaim their health, step into their power, and create lives of fulfillment and purpose. May the pages of this book inspire you to embark on a path of self-discovery and transformation, radiating wellness and empowerment in every aspect of your life.

With heartfelt gratitude and unwavering belief in your potential,

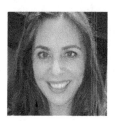

—Dr. Claire Zammit
Founder, The Institute for Woman-Centered Coaching, Training & Leadership

Preface

I met and was drawn to Beatriz the first day of medical school when I helped her carry her bags into our dorm, Bard Hall, at Columbia University's College of Physicians and Surgeons. About eight months later, my best friend, Brad, was visiting from law school. Brad asked me whether we should invite her to come with us to see a movie when dance rehearsal for Pippin, the play Beatriz and I were in together, was canceled. "Don't even try to ask her," I responded. "There are always six or more guys after her. You're just going to get shut down." But Brad didn't think we had anything to lose since he was going back to law school. He figured if she said no, we could both still see the movie.

Fortunately, Beatriz said yes and off we went to see the movie *Breaker Morant*, a fine Australian film. Afterwards, we headed to a bar to discuss the movie and really enjoyed sharing ideas together. Later that night, Brad asked me, "Why don't you ask Beatriz out?" I didn't want to be one of the guys who were annoying her, I explained, like another gnat around a lightbulb.

Later that Spring during another play rehearsal, I overheard Beatriz mention her upcoming birthday. As the date approached, I learned that she had scheduled a series of commitments throughout the day. Finally, I saw my chance! I wrote her a note, inviting her to join me to celebrate her birthday in my room in Bard Hall at 11pm "with some, alas domestic, champagne?" Happily for me, she said yes. Those early "yesses" led to marriage, raising a family and continuing to keep our love alive through continuing to date for more than 42 years. I continue to be inspired by and learn from Beatriz every day.

I've had the privilege of witnessing the gestation and birth of *Mind Body Secrets*. The book is a culmination of both Beatriz's personal and professional journey over many years. This is not a book filled with gimmicks, exaggerations or lies. Instead, you are receiving the authentic evolution of both Beatriz as a woman and a physician. If you seek wellness, as she did when she was an overweight and depressed teenager, then this book includes Beatriz's personal struggles and triumphs and her professional insights and discoveries. If you seek a road map, then this book will take you along a true, evidence-based, and expansive path. The book is a user manual to aid all of us to comprehend the significance of our shared ancestral biological adaptations when many of us in the developed world live with food abundance.

Beatriz is an outstanding scientist, and, as a fellow physician and scientist, I have shared in the joy of her original scientific discoveries. She wrote the definitive paper on low sodium levels in the blood following pituitary gland surgery. She helped characterize the water channel in the kidney that became the basis for a new class of medication. I was fortunate to travel to Paris with her while we were pregnant with our first child. There, she presented her original work on appetite and satiety, proving pathways between the vagus nerve and the brain, at the Society for the Study of Ingestive Behavior. That work on oxytocin, decades later, again became the basis for a new use of a hormone to help regulate appetite. In another study, she discovered how the brain changes hormonal pulse releases when women are thin to decrease ovarian follicle growth. This evolutionary adaptation helps humans not get pregnant when there is a famine.

Beatriz's ability to absorb science has helped her when she reads basic science articles and uses this knowledge to anticipate new approaches for taking care of her patients. For example, she used metformin and weight loss to help reverse diabetes a decade before this became standard care. Her mind allows her to peer into the future. Among her many talents, she is also a world-class thyroidologist.

Beatriz came to the United States with a good education, a strong family, and a powerful attitude. People who meet Beatriz usually don't know that when she first arrived in this country as a Cuban immigrant, she was not treated well at all. The American foods she ate upon arrival did not help her go through puberty well. Instead, she gained weight and became obese. She also became less physically active because her family wanted to protect her from the people who might further mistreat her and cause her harm. This combination of eating the Standard American Diet and less activity resulted in weight gain.

Beatriz struggled to learn English, fit in and feel a sense of belonging, and lose the weight she had gained. Her curiosity, determination, drive, and grit allowed her to begin her own journey of transformation. She explored and uncovered the root causes and solutions to overcome disliking herself and her excess weight. Jungian psychotherapy, meditation, Buddhist studies, and other research enabled Beatriz to heal many of her childhood demons and the negative voices within. She has maintained a healthy weight since we were married 40 years ago. We typically enjoy coffee in the morning and one meal at dinner each day. As this book teaches, experiencing a little hunger daily is beneficial to our health and helps keep us young.

One of the significant learning adventures Beatriz and I enjoyed together occurred in the mid '90s. We traveled to California to learn Mind-Body Medicine and Ayurveda with Deepak Chopra. Later, we traveled to Goa, India for the advanced chakra and sutra-based meditation training course "Seduction of Spirit." This was transformative for both of us. What we learned together inspired me and became the basis for how I pause for meditation in the middle of the day. This ten-minute practice reboots my mind and allows me to become refreshed and ready for my afternoon patients. Awareness of how the body and mind work together also helps me in my orthopaedic practice.

Beatriz integrated the insights and wisdom that emerged from her transformational journey into her services as a physician. She remained committed to and furthered her quest to ongoing learning to serve even more people by founding Lotus, The Educational Center for Integrative Healing and Wellness, in Connecticut. Lotus provided many integrative and complementary healing modalities: chiropractic, massage therapy, myofascial therapy, Polarity, EMDR, naturopathy, hypnotherapy, hospice, and others. During the fifteen years that this group met monthly, we all learned and developed trust in the healing intentions and methods of our fellow healers to whom we had not been exposed in our earlier medical training.

Beatriz provides exceptional support to her patients because of her vast and impressive accumulation of medical knowledge. She is an expert diagnostician. She understands medical and hormone diseases thoroughly. She also knows when such diseases are not the problem. Unlike most medical doctors, however, Beatriz is able to then tackle her patients' symptoms and ailments, whether physical, psychological or even soul distress. Her experiences have taught her that all three domains need to be addressed: mind, body and spirit. I believe that *Mind Body Secrets* will take you and every reader further along the path of transforming your health and wellness more than any book you've ever read.

The journey of transformation requires effort. When we wish to make change, we must persist through the inevitable challenges and difficulties that emerge with letting go of old patterns and establishing new ones. *Mind Body Secrets* will help you much more if rather than just reading and studying the book, you also view and listen to the guided meditations Beatriz has embedded at the end of each chapter. Further, to concretely set and reach your own goals, buy a notebook and write answers to the questions at the end of each chapter in the "Journaling for Transformation" sections.

Beatriz has taken all she has learned to a new level in the writing of this book. *Mind Body Secrets* offers a true distillation of the essential essence of what Beatriz knows. If you are earnest about wanting to keep yourself out of the medical care system, transform your life and your health for the better, and understand how to live with genuine health in the contemporary world, then you need to study what's in this book. These truths are not going to change. Translating what you learn in *Mind Body Secrets* into action will require dedication. *This book teaches all of the ways that self-care and tending to our needs is the path to freedom, health, connection to others and longevity.* Your commitment and efforts will lead you along the path to a healthier and more vibrant life for the remainder of your days.

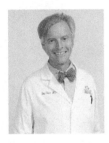

—Eric Jon Olson, MD
Fellow, American Academy of Orthopaedic Surgeons, President, Waterbury Orthopaedic Associates, Waterbury, CT

Introduction

In the early 1990s pressures erupted when my husband, Eric, also a physician, was called overseas to serve our country. Professional requirements of running a unit at the National Institute of Health were already significant. The sudden strain of juggling my medical career with managing our home and parenting our two precious young daughters without Eric's help impacted my immune system. I was diagnosed and struggled through mononucleosis. My body and head ached. High fevers and chills were uncontrollable. I sank into debilitating exhaustion. The sliver of stability I was barely holding onto was slipping from my grasp.

I had to do something because my two little girls were depending on me. My team and staff at the NIH were depending on me. So, what do you think I decided? What was the most scientific choice a doctor like me could make to prevent the ship of her life from sinking?

I made one simple decision. A decision that the average individual might not believe could help. A decision that brings chuckles to the doctors to whom I lecture on the topics of disenfranchisement and burnout. A decision that astonishes even me.

I called a nail salon and scheduled an appointment for a manicure.

During those 40 or so minutes at the nail salon, something happened that surprised me. I had not been touched in so long with my husband gone, that I didn't realize how a simple hand massage and color painted on my nails could bring life back to my ailing body. Something so small—a single decision to tend to myself and the kindness and services provided by the nail technician—helped me to rise up to more effectively manage the demands of my career and taking care of my daughters.

I have worked with thousands of patients over the course of my medical career who want to rise up through illness and disease, excess weight and the various stresses of our contemporary world. They come to me focused on their physical well-being and transforming numbers on the scale, lab levels and their clothing sizes. I can relate to my patients. As a young woman, I immigrated to America from Cuba and gained weight from eating the standard American diet. I struggled, like many of my patients, with excess weight and obesity. I yearned to lose weight, wear a smaller clothing size, and eat fewer calories. I was focused on the physical, not initially understanding the importance of aligning the mind with the body.

As an integrative medicine physician and an individual who desires to live a healthy and vibrant life, I have come to believe that the mind and body work as a unit. When we align our mind and body we can enter and proceed down the path of realizing optimal health and vitality. In *Mind Body Secrets* I offer information and stories that synthesize over 40 years of experience, research, academic training, and medical expertise.

But I continue to wrestle with a challenging question: when so many of us are focused on our physical health, how can I make it clear that we absolutely must start with the mind? Becoming conscious of how our mind is wired is critical to achieving and sustaining health. I have witnessed in myself and my patients that the more we understand our ancestral biology, a biology that has not changed to keep up with our constantly changing world, the more we develop the capacities to start and sustain health transformation.

This is why I begin the book providing necessary information about the mind. I continually refer to the mind throughout the book to urge you to become aware of the existential clash between our ancestrally wired need for biological survival and how these needs can be met by us in our current modern environment. Many of our physical behaviors, mindsets, and reactions are ancestrally wired. The body's biology, therefore, responds to current life situations as if living in earlier rather than contemporary times. Hundreds of thousands of years of scarcity and famines, coupled with the drive to survive and reproduce, created food and lifestyle patterns for those particular times.

Our current reality differs from ancestral times. We don't face scarcity to the extent we did even 100 years ago. However, we are still wired to over-consume as if preparing for famine or food scarcity, even when there is food abundance. In addition, the body deals with different ingredients in processed foods that negatively impact our metabolism and minds. Further confusing our metabolic and hormone systems is the constant presence of light in our homes and from our computers. In the past, the night-day light cycle influenced our circadian and hormonal rhythms, and we benefited from the healing properties of sleep. Now we are sleep-deprived and less physically active, which prevents us from effectively dealing with the overwhelming distractions and stresses of modern-day life. Disconnected from the needs of our bodies, we live in our heads and absorb the relentless persuasive messaging and information bombarding us to do, achieve and have more. We feel inadequate. We worry there is not enough time to satisfy these ancestrally-wired biologic drives to measure up and conform to the crushing rhythms of our current culture.

Living this type of life is incompatible with true health. Our ancestral wiring for survival keeps working as if we are living in the past, but we're living in the here and now, in contemporary environments. As a result, our hormones, metabolism, and neurotransmitters go haywire. This mismatch results in biological and cognitive dissonance, resulting in disease, soul distress, and a lack of wellness in multiple domains of our lives, not just our physical health. We risk and are currently experiencing medical catastrophe and outrageous medical costs. We are aging faster and suffering from early disabilities.

I was motivated to write *Mind Body Secrets* because, like so many of us, I endured the loss of friends, families, and patients during the pandemic. I began to fear that I might be a casualty of Sars-Covid 2.

What if I died without sharing key knowledge to protect and heal this and next generations? I knew that I would deeply regret not sharing the valuable scientific and spiritual truths that I have learned during more than 40 years of personal experiences and professional research and expertise as a doctor. I felt a sense of urgency, a deep calling, and a mission, to provide more people than I can possibly treat with the knowledge to remain well despite these and future changing times.

Another reason I knew I needed to write this book is that we are living in critical times. Despite many of us living in a developed world, we are suffering from illnesses and diseases that may be epigenetically transferred to the next generations, making it increasingly harder to avoid or reverse diseases. While many of us tend to blame ourselves for our health challenges, I wish to emphasize that it's not our fault. We have turned to mainstream medicine, which is dedicated to treating and alleviating the symptoms of illnesses and diseases rather than addressing the root problems we face. The knowledge, insights, and stories I bring to you are not part of mainstream medicine. I have titled this book *Mind Body Secrets* because I desire to share information that is less accessible or simply not available. The new insights and knowledge in the pages ahead will help us address and solve the health problems we face, individually and collectively. We all deserve to know about the mind-body-spirit pathways available to us that, if understood, will empower us to heal, to prevent and reverse illness, to age slower and more successfully, to cultivate vibrancy, and to live long and meaningful lives.

And so, dear reader, I bring to you a road map, a health and vitality map, that contains the secrets, the less available information than what you typically receive while visiting your primary care provider. Start where you are right now and use this map to begin your journey, explore new possibilities, develop new potentialities, and embrace your wholeness. You can and will transform your health with dignity and wisdom. You can and will empower yourself in all domains of your life using this map. Take one step at a time and nurture and manage your mind, your body, and your soul.

The figure below summarizes the knowledge and skills you need to move from one step to the next. We begin with the mind. When we manage the ways of the mind, we access unimaginable power. When we understand and care for the mind, we can more effectively care for and nourish the body. Learning to appreciate and honor our mind and body is enhanced by connecting to our spirit. Tending to higher levels of consciousness opens us up to expansive possibilities and results.

While you may be tempted to use this book as a guide or self-care manual, you can maximize your transformation by starting and maintaining a journal using the prompts at the end of each chapter. Align your mind, body and spirit by using the meditations embedded throughout the book. Keep an open mind and a compassionate and patient attitude toward yourself and others as you evolve. Remember that vision and consistent action will move you through the journey. I'll see you on the other side.

Mind Body Secrets Map

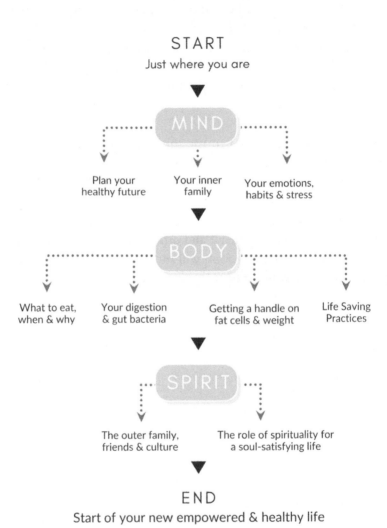

START
Just where you are

▼

MIND

Plan your
healthy future

Your inner
family

Your emotions,
habits & stress

▼

BODY

What to eat,
when & why

Your digestion
& gut bacteria

Getting a handle on
fat cells & weight

Life Saving
Practices

▼

SPIRIT

The outer family,
friends & culture

The role of spirituality for
a soul-satisfying life

▼

END
Start of your new empowered & healthy life

Figure 1. The Mind Body Secrets Map to Health. Start
just where you are. Take the steps through the journey and
transform the quality of your life and your health.

Care of The Mind

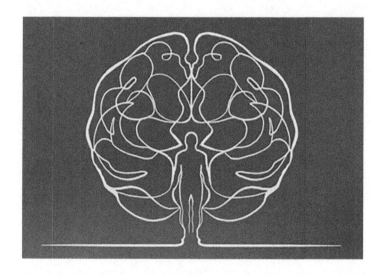

Chapter 1

Envision Your Healthy Future

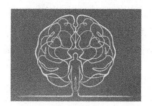

Transformation is Possible

Allow me to take you on a transformational journey to envision and create the vibrant life you deserve. What would it mean for you if you felt truly well in your body all the time? What would you enjoy the most? How would changes in your health and well-being serve you, your family, your work, and the world around you?

Most of us don't ask ourselves these questions. Most of us have a limited vision of our health and our lives. We create a vision of what could be from our current experiences and reality. Sometimes it is hard to envision how we could be healthier and have more energy. Many of us become complacent. We may associate things like weight gain or particular ailments with getting older. We don't question if this is the way it has to be. And some of us stop believing that change is possible because we have tried but never reached our goals.

I am here to disrupt this kind of limited thinking. In the past I, too, suffered from such thinking. I came to the United States as a child from Cuba. I was the oldest daughter of highly educated parents. Though educated, my family had very little money. I struggled with adjusting and fitting in as an immigrant. I indulged in the affordable standard American diet and became sick. I had negative thoughts around my looks and sense of belonging. I sometimes thought that I was not welcome. I felt insecure and invisible.

With time, I went on to become a doctor, a wife, and a mother; I celebrate that I am a creative, transformed, and empowered woman. New awareness and curiosity allowed me to move beyond my limited perceptions and beliefs. I learned new skills and ways of being that gave traction to sustainably achieve vibrant health. The same is possible for you. You can transform and improve any domain of your life.

My Story

Shortly after my family first arrived in America, I struggled. I was the subject of discrimination because of my foreign appearance and poor English skills. Strangers called me "spic." I also became an obese teenager because I was less active and consumed the American diet. I became unrecognizable to myself in the mirror. I received negative comments from my own family, and others, for my inability to manage my weight and my new "fatso" appearance.

Other people's negative reactions and my psychological reaction to them, combined with my sense of not belonging in this new country, fractured my sense of wholeness. I suffered the consequences in my body and my mind. I felt unhappy and deeply frustrated with how I looked and felt.

My family watched as I tried a variety of ways to lose weight, hoping one would work for me. I exercised to *Workout Starring Jane Fonda*, a popular video, to *feel the burn*. I experimented with a variety of diets. I tried laxatives, supplements, even salted ace bandages wrapped around my hips, butt and thighs. I even resorted to bulimia, which only added another burden to my anguish.

Despite my efforts, none of these provided lasting solutions. I was surprised that nothing seemed to work. I felt helpless, embarrassed, and disempowered. I felt a deep sense of shame and *not-enoughness* for not being able to solve this paradox: With all my intelligence, I could not uncover the secrets to losing weight and fixing my broken self-esteem.

What I didn't know then is that my self-perception affected how I showed up in the world. I didn't believe that I belonged or that I was worthy of being seen or heard. I was unaware that my weight gain and inability to lose it was driven by my new lifestyle in America and old biological ancestral adaptations that had evolutionarily been developed thousands of years ago for humans to survive and reproduce.

I was fortunate, though, that despite the limiting thoughts in my head and excess weight in my body, I was motivated to learn enough to become healthier and help others who suffered similarly. A career in medicine could perhaps help me answer the questions that had been haunting me for so long: *How can I restore my health? How can I feel comfortable in my own skin again?*

In medical school at Columbia University, I met my beautiful husband, Eric. A former collegiate athlete and runner at Princeton, he encouraged me to try running. He taught me to jog and years later to run marathons, which we did together during our residencies after medical school. I never knew I had that in me.

The demands of my medical school schedule and dancing and choreographing for the Bard Hall Players, our theater group, distracted me and increased my activities in the evening. Between the studying, the school lectures and labs, and the extra-curricular activities, I ended up routinely having just one meal a day. It turned out that as a petite woman who struggled with obesity earlier in life, this pattern worked well for me. By the time I was a third-year medical student and married Eric, I was a normal-weight person. As I write this book, I have been the same weight for almost 40 years.

Early on, I did not understand the power of movement and the fact that we don't need an excess of food to be well and thrive. Becoming an endocrinologist allowed me to understand how hormones work and how lifestyle, stress, and fat cells interact with our metabolism. I learned that our ancestral survival biology evolved to prevent us from losing weight. And eventually, I learned about limiting beliefs—thoughts, opinions, convictions, and stories that we regard as absolute truths that hold us back, and how these beliefs sabotage our efforts to sustainably transform our lives for the better.

In my particular medical school, we students were encouraged to receive psychotherapy, because a life unexamined was not worth living. Receiving these services benefited me. I, like many of you, have experienced losses and disappointments. I was traumatized by childhood uncertainties of safety for my family while we were in the formidable process of leaving a communist regime and immigrating to another country. I have post-traumatic stress disorder (PTSD) and hyper-alertness as a result of these early life experiences. My body can easily jump into primitive survival alarm mode at any time when my mind senses danger or uncertainty.

Since medical school, I have continued on the path of personal development. I have benefited from years of Jungian psychotherapy, Buddhist philosophy, and a meditation practice to calm my fears, fight-flight-freeze stress-activated system, and perfectionism. Over time, I have learned to meet my needs and practice self-compassion. I continue to take a little time to stop, breathe and be so I can connect to higher awareness, my spirit, inspiration, and creativity. When I engage in these simple practices, I reboot the computer of my brain, and I offer my energy and gifts with abundance and less reservation.

Developing a nurturing relationship with myself was crucial to discovering that I am whole, just as I was at the beginning when I was born, before all the cultural and social demands, persuasions and distractions led to behaviors, beliefs, and physical and emotional changes that took me away from my health and my truth. I have actively transformed my wellness and health. I have revitalized other domains of my life–my family life, my career, my friendships. I have walked the path of personal and professional transformation, and I have helped my patients do the same. I am inviting you to join me and create a new vision for yourself and your wellness, or in any domain of your life you'd like to change. You *can* transform your life for the better.

Transformation & Helpful Terms

Transformation is a profound process that brings our whole being in alignment with our potentialities. Our perceptions and beliefs change and spur progress in multiple domains of our life: physical, emotional, psychological, spiritual, relational, and financial.

Transforming our health is a journey. There are no fast or gimmicky ways to do this. The work of personal transformation is about deeply seeing the space between where we are and where we want to be. We all yearn to go someplace that is better, like the positive setting of the afterlife in *The Good Place*, the fabulous Netflix series. We seek a higher level of being, of wellness, but we can only start where we are, in the present moment, and we often find it hard to leave and get to the place or state-of-being we yearn for.

Helpful Terms

Wellness combines many domains: spiritual, physical, mental, and psychological. Wellness includes the conscious awareness that you are comfortable in your body and safe in your space.

Health is the absence of physical and psychological disease.

Well-Healthy combines the concepts of wellness and health.

The Challenges of Transformation

Many of us have the experience of wanting to make changes in our lives. We want to start exercising, but after two weeks we stop. We want to lose weight, but after a few weeks we get discouraged by setbacks, and then relapse to where we were when we started. We want to have love in our lives, but at some level we are afraid and don't want to be hurt again, so when love comes, we let it go or push it away. We want to prevent an illness, yet we continue unhealthy habits. We want financial prosperity, but we continue to spend more so our debt grows. Many of us get fatigued from cycles of trying and failing, and doubt that change is truly possible. I understand this deeply.

Transformation is uncomfortable. Our ancestral brain, the part of the brain made for survival, struggles to make changes because we are wired to maintain ourselves and the world around us to be safe and stable. We are conditioned by culture and social networks to maintain our current identity and habits, even if these keep us unwell. Maintaining the status quo is part of an ancestral system that keeps us surviving but not thriving. There are biological and ancestral reasons for this, so to some extent, it's not all our fault. Once we know how to handle these survival-wired adaptations, we can actually take responsibility for getting around them. In addition to repeating ancestral patterns even when they don't serve us, social forces can hold us back. Family, friends, and colleagues may express their discomfort with the changes we are making, preferring our old, less-well identity. The need for belonging and acceptance may offset our desire for change.

Our inability to reach our goals can cause frustration, shame and other negative feelings that trigger unconscious patterns such as hiding and isolating ourselves. This keeps us stuck where we are. We are unable to function at our highest potential because we don't have the bandwidth. We are like an eight-cylinder engine where not all the cylinders are functioning well. Why is that?

First and primarily, we fail to achieve our health goals in the various domains of our life because we lack awareness of our own needs and how to tend to them. These include the needs of our body, mind, and spirit. Most of us have not acquired the tools and skills necessary to care for these entities of our being. We may be unaware of how the body hangs on to old ways of being and how our culture and friends influence our behavior and interfere with our ability to make sustainable changes to our lives. This lack of knowledge keeps us unfulfilled. When we have awareness of the physical, mental, and spiritual dimensions of our journey towards health, as well as an understanding of the forces that will need to be overcome along this journey, we develop our capacity to make lasting changes. Transformation begins with a conscious intention to change our behavior and consistent, small, steady steps to get there.

The second obstacle to achieving our health goals is that we source power from outside of ourselves. We assume that our problems can be solved by quick fixes, the internet, or by seeing experts who offer advice or prescribe pills, not questioning whether or not the advice or prescriptions are connected to our true needs and values. We may even sense that these professionals have low expectations of what we might achieve. These internalized assumptions and our own lack of awareness hinder us from seeing our potential to be and feel better. We cannot see the possibility that we can access our inherent healing capacity by making new informed decisions and taking actions that are more aligned to what our body truly needs to achieve our highest health.

The third hindrance to reaching our health goals is that we are not able to connect to a motivation that is powerful enough to overcome our setbacks and limitations. In my experience, there are three motivators that ignite lasting change: 1) Finding what it is costing us to remain unwell and learning how to reverse or prevent the problem; 2) finding an inner reason for change that is connected to our core values; 3) and/or being inspired by someone that we identify with who has been successful in their personal change. These internal motivators energize and enable transformation. When these elements and persistent actions are directed toward your vision, success is inevitable.

An Individual & Integrative Approach to Transformation

Transformation is a very individual process because we all have unique situations, needs, and challenges. Transformation requires an integrative approach that embraces our complexity. We must honor the essential interactions between our mind and body. We must integrate our spiritual energy and soulful experiences. Developing a conscious and connected relationship with ourselves is central to the process, as is allowing curiosity about and compassion toward ourselves. We must be willing to challenge old ideas to create actions that support our nascent healthy identity.

The Steps to Transformation Wheel

Through my work with patients and as a transformational leader, I've learned that there are logical steps that we can take to improve our quality of life. Taking the steps along the path helps us to shift our current limiting mindsets and unhelpful behaviors into more empowered mindsets and actions that will support the healthy future self we seek. I learn best when I can visualize a process so I created the Transformation Steps wheel, shown in Figure 2, which shows eight steps to transformation. It is reassuring and motivating for our brain to know where we are along the way to making the intended, sustainable change. Knowing that there are eight steps keeps us focused on the task, even if we don't know what the ultimate outcome will be. Further, if something happens that slows our journey along the way we know where to hop back on again. When we accomplish each step of the journey, we have an opportunity to celebrate our efforts. Once you understand the steps and dynamics of change, you have power.

The Steps to Transformation

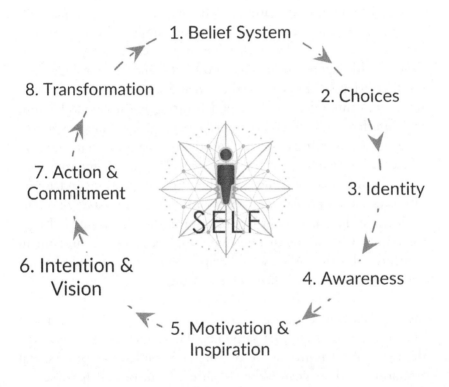

1. Belief System

8. Transformation

2. Choices

7. Action &
Commitment

3. Identity

6. Intention &
Vision

4. Awareness

5. Motivation &
Inspiration

SELF

Figure 2. The Steps to Transformation Wheel

The Eight Steps to Transformation

Step 1 - The current **Belief System**. This is the place where we start. Who we are and what we believe about ourselves is a distillation of our family, our upbringings, our sense of poverty or wealth, our ethnic backgrounds, prevalent culture, our past experiences and traumas. All these things create the sense of what we are about, our sense of belonging, our yearnings, what we believe we are capable of, how we manage and express—or not—our emotions and stress, and how safe or empowered we feel. These influences also affect our views about health, aging, spirituality, prosperity, and relationships. Our mindset (what we think about things), and setpoints (what we think we can or cannot do), can be useful at fitting-in early on in life, but may interfere with our ability to make sustainable changes as adults. A key aspect of trying to make a substantive change is to understand where we personally are at the start, *now*. We can become conscious of our current state of being and beliefs by being curious and asking ourselves questions. Are we happy with our current state of affairs in different domains of our life, like our health? If we could change something, what would that be? Why would a change in this domain make us feel better? What would help us move forward and what are perceivable blockages to making this change?

Step 2 - Choices. The actions and choices we make are a direct result of self-beliefs and cultural setpoints. These include diet, lifestyle, the types of relationships we pursue, and the level of professional aspirations and life goals we've visualized. Some of us believe we can do anything, take risks and go beyond our comfort zones to grow. And some of us have been hurt, feel unseen, disenfranchised, or held back by cultural or societal ideas. As a result, we may believe that the world is not safe, that what we do doesn't matter, that we don't deserve to aim high or have better, or that we don't trust or believe in ourselves. In this state of contraction, we have limited vision and limited possibility for growth and change, and our choices are also limited or unhelpful. We may choose the wrong foods, the wrong partners, or lose opportunities. This mindset prevents us from making more thoughtful choices that are aligned with our deeper, higher values as adults.

Therefore, we must ask ourselves, what choices are we making, and do they really support who we are now and our future goals? Is it possible that the way we perceive ourselves limits our capacity to make mature choices as adults in varied aspects of life? Are we creating healthy wellness behaviors or not? Can we believe the story that our brain has been giving us?

For example, when I came from Cuba, we were poor. We picked up furniture from the street and my mother and I reupholstered it. Because I grew up with a poverty-conscious mindset, I always thought I would have used furniture. It took years for me to believe that I could actually buy new furniture. This is how our early mindset and upbringing can limit our possibilities and choices when we become adults.

Step 3 - Our current **Identity** is shaped by old actions and choices that are made by our current belief system, limiting setpoints, and unchallenged beliefs. This identity defines how we show up. It may be keeping you stuck where you are and preventing your yearnings from becoming a reality. For example, you may want to lose weight as an adult, but as a younger, thinner person, you were sexually abused. Perhaps you gained weight as a protective mechanism to avoid this abuse again. So now as an adult, you lose weight with effort. Maybe when some random person makes a move, touches you, or comments on your appearance, you are put on the alert based on your prior experience. This previously traumatized younger-inner part of you that is trying to protect you, the adult, from harm, emotionally triggers a desire for doughnuts and high-carb meals. The past trauma experience sabotages your adult efforts to lose or maintain weight. Most of us are unaware of these inner interactions happening within our minds. Unless you understand this paradigm, you may continue to have difficulty trying to change something that has protected you in the past. Being curious as to why we sabotage ourselves and gaining new awareness unlocks the process.

Step 4 - Awareness comes from new knowledge and understanding. Awareness creates a higher state of consciousness that gives us more possibility and expands our choices. This is how we begin to challenge old assumptions about ourselves and others. When we do this, we can give new meaning to old stories. When we see things in a different light, we have a greater potential to bring our yearnings for change to fruition.

Step 5 - The **Motivation and Inspiration** to create change. External motivations, such as someone paying you to lose weight, are less effective than internal motivations for change. Internal motivations are more powerful because they give meaning to life or are linked to things that we value (being with family, creating memories, helping family or society, etc.). For example, you want to be more fit so make changes in your busy schedule, or lose weight so you can be part of a great hiking group that raises money for something you believe in, or because you want to travel and be active with your children and grandchildren on the next vacation. Being inspired by someone we identify with is also a strong motivator for change.

Step 6 - The **Intention** to create a new **vision**. Visualizing ourselves as healthy or having achieved our goal can help us stay focused and succeed. Athletes do this all the time. Can you visualize yourself feeling well in your body? Feeling strong and flexible? Entering a room where you are welcomed and valued just because you are your authentic self? Fitting into your beautiful wardrobe? Being energetic in your job? When you do this, you are visualizing the person you will be after creating the change. Visualizing this future new, healthy, and well identity helps us create a horizon to aim for and to activate our intention to create it. This is where we begin thinking about how we can create the environment to succeed and what skills we will need. Who can support us? How can we learn to actively block negative self-talk, devaluing comments, and perfectionism that puts us in a non-possibility mindset?

Step 7 - The *new* **Actions** and the **Commitment** taken to support lasting change. We can have a lot of intentions and desires, but without taking action it all becomes an illusion. I have found that planning and putting myself on the calendar is essential. We need to commit to showing up for ourselves and our planned exercise or activity. When we show up and do what we say we are going to do, we develop confidence. We can see that we have resilience and grit to stay on task, even if some days things don't work out as we had planned. It is helpful to have a positive attitude and make whatever action we are doing fun. Persistence, planning, and practice create, in time, new habits which match the new *well-healthy* identity. In Step 7, these are integrated and grounded in the new identity.

Step 8 - The **Transformation** has occurred: We have learned to evolve from where we were to where we are. We now show up differently as our new well-healthy identity. We have created new patterns of thoughts and ideas about ourselves and what we are capable of. New habits are established and are part of who we are *now*. We can re-enter Step 1 with a new mindset and belief system that supports and sustains the changes made.

The **self**, or our inner being, is at the core of all of these outer transformational influence domains. This is the place where we can reach our authentic being, our essence, our aliveness and wholeness. Within the self exists the connection to spirit-energy and the soulful experience of life. The self holds our unique gifts and talents and capacity to access possibilities within ourselves and beyond our comprehension. The ability to heal ourselves is within this space, bringing us to our wholeness. The more we connect to our self, explore our beliefs and actions, ways of being and our true needs, the more authentic our existence becomes, and the more we are able to accomplish and give to others.

Case Study: Barbara's Story

The following case study illustrates the steps of transformation using the Transformation Steps. Barbara is a woman in her early fifties who has been trying to lose weight for decades. When I met and learned about her situation, I could clearly see that she cycled through steps one through three over and over and was stuck in a non-possibility about her situation. Her belief system and actions perpetuated a limited self-identity that prevented her from taking off weight. She believed that like many women she would retain some extra weight after the birth of each of her children. She accepted the cultural idea that losing weight after menopause would be difficult. She was aware of healthy food and exercise choices; she was even successful at losing weight for some period of time, but then she would revert to her old weight, or slightly higher, the following year.

When she regained the weight, she tried even harder to lose weight and succeeded for periods of time with the use of weight-loss medications. Invariably, she would stop the medication and regain the weight. Her husband, who did not have a weight issue and often cooked the house meals, could not understand why she just did not eat less or avoid unhealthy food. His feedback added to her sense of not-enoughness and low self-esteem.

Barbara felt ashamed of her inability to succeed at weight loss and believed she could only do so with diet pills that curbed her appetite, but she hated having to be dependent on them. She used high-calorie carbohydrate-rich foods to help her feel better—to soothe guilt she had for not maintaining a consistent exercise program and the anxiety about issues at home with her husband and children. She often rationalized that she was busy tending to the needs of her family. Over time, she lost the belief that she could help herself and felt locked in an inner jail.

At her annual doctor's visit, Barbara was informed that her fasting sugars and cholesterol were getting high. This new information catapulted her into step four of the Transformation Steps. The information from the doctor and the realization—*awareness*—that she could potentially develop diabetes and need cholesterol-lowering medicine for the rest of her life concerned her. Members of her extended family had diabetes and cancer. She feared that she could be heading in the same direction.

Shortly after learning this new information, she had lunch with a friend she had known for years, who, like her, carried excess weight. She could not believe the transformation in her friend. She was slim and filled with vitality. Her friend shared that what motivated her to take charge of her health, to lose weight and to make choices to enhance her energy, was preparing for the wedding of her child. She didn't want the permanent wedding pictures to reflect her overweight self.

Then and there, Barbara shifted into step five of the Transformation Steps—the *motivation and inspiration to change*. My patient clearly understood the physical consequences of her excess weight from the visit with her doctor. She also understood the potential psychological impact that permanent photos of her excess weight would create during the luncheon with her friend. You see, Barbara's child was engaged to be married the following year.

Motivated to create a new slimmer, healthier vision of herself and emboldened to reverse and prevent disease, Barbara entered steps five and six. She *created a vision* of how she wanted to look at her daughter's wedding, and in the memories created by photos on that day. She *committed to daily action*s to create a slimmer and healthier version of herself. She began to plan meals and make healthier food choices. She convinced her husband to cook with healthy ingredients, and she also prepared more of the meals. She purchased a rowing machine, which she used daily, increasing the time with each session. Gradually, Barbara saw changes in her body. The results showed up in her blood tests as well. Her sugar and cholesterol normalized. She was physically stronger and felt more confident as her innate sense of power to commit to transformation increased.

Part of step seven of the Transformation Steps is sustaining the new actions taken to support lasting change. Barbara was developing capacities to plan her day and meals more effectively. She was consistent in creating new habits to match the healthy vision she had established for herself. She was finally experiencing the success she had not achieved in the past and was proud of the work she had done to achieve this new healthier identity. At her daughter's wedding, she felt vibrant in her body and she treasured wearing her silky blue dress.

Barbara journeyed through each step of the Transformation Steps, including step eight. She experienced a complete *transformation* that she has sustained by developing new beliefs and behaviors to match her vision. Now, years later, she still rows, walks, or bikes most days, and if she misses a day, she plans for the next time that she can exercise. She now believes that exercise helps her deal with stress. She notes that she is calmer and more mindfully responsive to all around her. While she continues to nourish herself with healthy foods, she enjoys an occasional ice cream without berating herself. She knows an occasional treat will not sabotage her resolve to be healthy and treasure the woman she has become. Self-compassion is key for her.

Having cycled entirely through the Transformation Steps, Barbara returned to step one with *new beliefs* that continue to guide her to take *new actions* that support her *new healthy self-identity*. She is now ready to challenge her next limiting setpoint that holds her back in other domains of her life.

How about you? What is your experience with transformation? What are the dreams and desires you have translated into reality? What are your unrealized dreams and desires? Are you ready to experience the Transformation Steps?

My Loving-Kindness Wish for You

May you be open and curious to new possibilities.
May you truly see yourself being healthy and well.
May you know that it is possible to achieve visions
with awareness and skills.

Meditation to Enhance Your Journaling

I recommend doing one of my short centering meditations before you explore the journaling prompts. Click on the link or scan the QR code for the meditation for this chapter. There will be a link and QR code for a meditation in each chapter that corresponds with that chapter.

Find a comfortable place to sit. Feel your hips and buttocks on the surface upon which you are sitting. Connect to your breath, feeling each breath enter and exit your body. As you breathe, feel the space around you. Become aware of your wise heartbeat. Allow your focus to be fully within you and connect to that part of you that shows up as your best. Invite that loving wise-adult self to be present within you.

Please scan the QR Code with your Smartphone
or follow this link: https://youtu.be/PQoGAnv75zk

Journaling for Transformation

Take time to journal and reflect on the following questions.

1. Envisioning a new level of wellness and health for yourself.
   - How do you define transformation?
   - What has prevented you from a lasting transformation? What holds you back?
   - How has this affected you emotionally? Physically? Spiritually?

2. What is one area of your health or other life domain (relationships, prosperity, spirituality) you would like to change?

   Use the Transformation Steps with curiosity and compassion for yourself to explore the domains of your life you'd like to improve.

   - Explore your current beliefs—cultural and family conditioning, past experiences, traumas.
   - Describe your current actions based on your beliefs.
   - What are the limitations of your current self-identity?
   - Explore your deeper yearnings and desires; create a new vision for yourself.
   - What new awareness do you have from reading this chapter?
   - What motivates and inspires you to fulfill these desires?

3. Intentions & Desires – what are your new intentions and desires for a healthy life? Can you visualize yourself being there?
   - How would you feel if you reached the best health goal for you?

- What new actions can you take consistently to support lasting change?
- Write about the transformation you desire as if you have achieved it. Describe what your new mindset and belief system would be.

Chapter 2

Your Inner Family

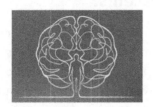

Mind-Body Systems & the Internal Family

Each one of us can harness our power and create the outcomes we desire by understanding the beauty and complexity of our mind, its relationship to the body, and getting to know our mind's *inner family system*. When the mind and body work together and our inner family system is embraced, we become more aware of how old ideas and outcomes can derail us from our desires and dreams. We can then reframe the present moment with more spaciousness and less stress. We can recognize new possibilities that help us manifest our mature desires.

Many of us struggle to be present in the here and now; we disrupt the mind-body's natural alignment by focusing on and worrying about the past and the future. We are triggered by people, places, and things. When this happens, we may experience a sudden burst of emotions. These emotions may arise from younger disenfranchised parts of ourselves, members of our inner family system, that rob us of higher conscious thinking, responses, and actions. We become vulnerable to poor decision-making and poor management of the stresses before us. We feel disconnected and alone. We are more susceptible to illness and aging faster.

We can transform deeply entrenched ancestral patterns, fears, and mindsets by better understanding the mind-body relationship, how our inner family system works, and adopting some empowering practices to support us through life's struggles.

What Are the Internal and Inner Family Systems?

While we have external or outer family members, such as parents and siblings, we also have internal family members. These internal family members are various parts of ourselves active in our consciousness. Some of these parts have not been fully integrated due to past trauma and they remain as younger, disenfranchised parts of ourselves. Our task is to become conscious of and integrate them to become more whole, taking care of them from the more mature adult part of ourselves when they are triggered.

This community of different parts of ourselves was first described by Dr. Richard Schwartz in his book, *The Internal Family System*. Individuals trained in Jungian psychology and trauma understand this concept because the focus of these therapies have to do with healing the inner child. Many of us intuitively know there are multiple parts of ourselves operating in our mind. This is not the same as a multiple personality psychiatric disorder or illness. It is simply a human condition, a fundamental truth, and influences our behavior in certain ways that can surprise us at times. This system is of utmost importance though rarely discussed in the medical community.

These younger parts of us that exist inside our mind influence how we show up in the world and whether we thoughtfully respond or emotionally react to situations and people. These younger parts shape our beliefs, mindset, values, sense of right and wrong, and behaviors. This inner community, the inner family system, creates our current identity, our sense of belonging and deservingness, and even our dreams and accomplishments. In this book, I will use the terms internal family system and inner family system interchangeably.

All of us have experienced some degree of trauma throughout our lives. For too many people, their childhoods include situational or ongoing trauma. Though every child deserves a safety system protecting them, tragically, not all children have this. Too many of us, when we were young, experienced devastating events before we even had the language or the maturity to describe and make sense of these situations.

We did not always have the necessary support to process these situations in productive ways. As a result, our younger selves disconnected and most likely made-up narratives that enabled us to survive the hurt and pain of those earlier moments. Without access to a mature and healthy adult, a wise self, to anchor us and provide a wise, safer, and more complete understanding of what had occurred, we (that younger part of us) disconnected from our wholeness. That younger part of ourselves developed immature protective mechanisms that may have helped us then but do not serve us now and may impair us as we grow older.

For example, if I lived in a home where my parents constantly yelled at or physically abused each other or me, I would not be able to make sense of the horror as a young child. An internal part of me might deal with the trauma by retreating, hiding in my room and eating chocolate because sweets soothe. I might pick my nails because doing so distracts me. If I were older, I might absorb myself in the world of media because doing so checks me out from the pain I cannot understand in front of me. I might join friends and drink and/or take drugs. I would be resorting to behaviors to suppress the pain and soothe myself, because I had not yet learned better ways of handling difficulties and coping. I would hopefully come to learn that these more protective ancestral reactions were not serving me and seek out the resources and support to develop my wiser self to create a successful and more joyful adult life.

As we understand our own internal family systems, we can come to accept and help disconnected younger parts of ourselves come back to wholeness. As they become seen and protected by our wise adult self, we increasingly disrupt old ways of functioning and empower ourselves to learn new, more mature ways of handling life's challenges.

My Story

I never went hungry when I lived in Cuba. However, from a young age, I knew about food rationing. We had to be mindful of having things last until the next time it was my family's turn to get their rations of coffee, rice, beans, soap, and other essentials. Seafood was never an option. And rarely steak. When we had steak, we cut it into many tiny morsels so everyone could have some. It was so deliciously prepared—pan-fried with onions and mixed with rice. Fidel Castro sometimes eliminated the Christmas holidays so we as a country could meet specific quotas in that working year. If Christmas occurred, we would get apples and canned strawberries.

In 2020, at the start of the SARS-CoV-2 pandemic, there was a sense that necessary household items would be unavailable. Most people began to hoard food and goods. I instead purchased our usual amounts of food and began to *ration* the portions of our meals. A few weeks into the pandemic, my husband and I, who are normal weight, began to lose weight, while some of my patients began to gain weight. Eric told me he had lost 6 pounds and asked if we should go back to larger portions. I had an unusual emotional reaction to this question. I got a stomach ache and nausea, which were uncommon for me. It was then that I became curious and took time to sit, breathe, and ask myself why I was behaving this way about our food management. Did it make sense for me to ration our portions when in fact, we still had the capacity to get food? What did I think would happen to us? I listened. I realized that my sudden urge to ration our food was rooted in childhood trauma. The seven-year-old of my inner family system had lived in fear of food scarcity. She had concerns and stomach pains. I could acknowledge the depth of her suffering from the viewpoint of the mature woman and mother I had become.

I held that young part of me with compassion, understanding where her fears came from. I reassured her that I would make sure that there was enough for everyone to eat, and reminded her that we were in America, where food is abundant beyond what we could have ever imagined possible in Cuba. I told her that there would be no lack and that we would all be fine. I thanked her for helping us be safe with her methods. My stomach pain slowly eased away. That evening I began serving normal portions of food again, and Eric's and my weight returned to normal in the following weeks. By becoming aware and curious about my emotional and physical reaction, I allowed myself to get in touch with a younger member of my inner family that was acting out to protect herself. Listening to her distress and fears, I embraced those feelings with love and support and restored a sense of wholeness that could provide a new meaning for the situation for her and me.

This is an example of the mind-body interactions we experience and how they are affected and emotionally informed by inner and younger parts of ourselves, or our inner family system.

Mind-Body Interactions

The body is a miraculous physical form created by molecules, cells, organs, and systems that work together and use energy to create and maintain life. The body is also part of the space we occupy physically and energetically in terms of what is seen and of the unseen surrounding atoms of energy that interact with the space around us. The brain controls every process in our physical body essential to our well-being and survival. It interprets our body's physical sensory experiences coming from the outside world. The body and brain work together as a unit sending signals back and forth to each other. For example, if the brain senses danger, our body's chemicals change to handle the stress. If while chopping onions we cut our finger, the brain receives the signal as pain and blood, and responds to this by creating physical actions to stop the bleeding. It learns to remember that sharp knives can cause pain. The brain is truly complex, such that it processes and creates logic from these inputs and helps generate the chemistry for the mind's thoughts, feelings, and behaviors.

Whereas the brain and body are physical, the mind is more of an abstract construct that exists within our more developed and contemporary brain. It involves consciousness, self-awareness, judgments and perceptions from our thoughts, and higher-level thinking. The mind is the conscious part of all of us that integrates thoughts, emotions, beliefs, and values. It also houses all the experiences and sensations we have had at different ages. More importantly, the mind interprets, judges, reacts and makes meaning of these experiences. This meaning-making at different levels of consciousness is important because it is linked to our ancestral survival needs. Our mind remembers where pleasure is and how to find it to soothe us, or where pain and horror exist and how to avoid it. The mind and body are interdependent. It is hard to believe that conventional medicine still considers that what happens in the mind does not affect the body or vice versa. From an integrative medicine perspective, the wellness of one depends on the other.

The more we understand how the brain and body work, the more empowered we can become to help it serve us. There is a more ancestral part of our brain (our limbic or reptilian brain) that reacts to events around us in primitive ways regarding survival, seeking pleasure and avoiding pain. And a more contemporary part of our brain, the frontal lobes that handle higher level thought, where discernment, judgment, and creativity lead to responsive rather than reactive decision-making and actions. If we are stressed or triggered by potential physical or emotional harm, the amygdala, the alarm system of our ancestral brain that perceives threats, turns on and activates other stress-responsive parts of the body. When the amygdala reacts, it disconnects us from our more advanced and conscious brain. Our frontal lobe is hijacked and shuts down. We can't respond rationally because we are in survival mode and are triggered into flight, fright, freeze. In these situations, we act from our ancestral brain's perspective. These may be appropriate or dysfunctional depending on what the current situation calls for in our modern world.

Sometimes our own thoughts, emotions from our inner family members, and unprocessed traumatic or painful experiences can be triggered, and our fears activate the amygdala's alarm system. This consequently causes physical symptoms, as it did for me during my pandemic food rationing period. Continuous or chronic primitive reactivity and its stress chemistry negatively impacts our overall health. By understanding and utilizing some inner family system practices, we can train our mind to learn new, more mature ways to respond, rather than react in primitive ways, to situations that trigger us.

An Integrative & Inner Family Systems Approach to Managing Weight

Weight gain and obesity are an epidemic. Weight loss is the biggest desire that my patients have and the area in which they most often struggle to succeed. I believe there are a few reasons for this, some of which are due to survival-set ancestral biology. Another important component is related to the younger members of our internal family that are active within us. Many of these younger parts act up in different ways, such as eating cookies to protect us from feeling our emotions or facing our daily stress or turmoil.

As adults now, we can feel surprised and wonder why we acted so angrily or why we ate in excess when we were not hungry. These behaviors are immature actions of our internal family member(s) trying to soothe and protect us. They are triggered within us by events, things, or people that frighten us and threaten our safety. They function to calm us and protect us, but they do it in a way that no longer serves our current, more mature reality and our goals to sustain weight loss. These ancestral-mind adaptations that we make to avoid pain and find pleasure clearly affect how we show up as adults and how we manage our yearnings and challenges.

We may begin to shame ourselves when we act out or behave in strange ways that are inconsistent with our current maturity and values, particularly if we don't understand or know how to control our behavior. We may criticize ourselves, thinking that we can shame ourselves into better action. We might say, "you're so stupid, you don't follow through, you're bad, you're not wanted." These derogatory comments are heard by our younger inner parts and reinforce their sense that they are exiled and remain unloved and disconnected. Negativity, self-deprecating comments, and perfectionism are the destroyers of possibility, potential, and joy. The routine use of these derogatory conversations with ourselves keeps us jailed and impotent. Derogatory self-conversations can alter neural pathways related to ways of thinking about ourselves and the world, robbing us of our power, motivation, and self-trust. When these new neural networks get established, they can impair our ability to be our best self in this lifetime.

How can we retrain our brains to consistently access our innate wise-adult self to create a new self-identity that is empowered and filled to the brim with wellness?

We can start by learning a simple centering practice to connect to the central wiser part of ourselves, which enables us to access a higher level of thought. We can learn to befriend our younger selves and respond to our ancestral reactions without judgment. To access our wisdom, we start by taking two to five-minute timeouts to connect to our breath, feel ourselves sitting in a chair with our feet touching the ground, and physically sense our bodies. Breathing practices are more clearly described in the journaling section of this chapter.

When we center ourselves like this, we learn to practice the virtue of curiosity. We can ask ourselves, "What am I really feeling?" We learn to listen without judgment to what is happening within ourselves, asking our wisest self to come out and serve as the adult in the room who can nurture and tend to the needs of the inner child that has made its presence known.

A deeper understanding of our internal family members also allows us the possibility to exercise more kindness to ourselves and stop the negative self-talk and self-deprecation that keeps us stuck in non-possibility. This is especially relevant when we think about the fact that these younger parts of us are individually acting to protect us but doing so in a manner we no longer want nor even need.

If we don't learn how to access the mature, wiser part of ourselves, it is like living in a house run by young children, with no adult present. In contrast, when we invite our wiser selves to honor the younger and disenfranchised inner family members and make them feel that they belong, something within shifts. This gives us our wholeness and our integrity, and from that place we can do so much more.

Understanding the sacred responsibility your wiser self has to comfort your inner child will reduce the number of cookies you consume, because you, the adult, will take initiative to lovingly address past traumas that are triggering overeating. This will bring you closer to your weight goals.

Steps to Transform Old Beliefs to New Beliefs

Figure 3 shows the process that empowers us to transform old beliefs into new beliefs. Here we are focusing on the first three steps of the Transformation Steps wheel in Chapter One. Notice that the inside of the triangle consists of the wise self. That's us—you and me. Our inner self, or the central essence of who we are, is always pure, whole, worthy, and good. However, this is often not what people see. As we grow, things happen, and we develop ways of being—our outer identity, protective personas, or self-branding—that make us fit in better with others and culture.

So, in fact, what others see is how we show up in the world, our **Current Identity**: how we dress, how we act, how we manage life and relationships, what we value, etc. Our current identity, therefore, is impacted by our life experiences with others like our family, friends, and foes and by our prevailing culture, religion, education, traumas, etc. Our current identity can evolve as we develop new knowledge, awareness, and skills. Current identity can also remain stagnant or can be controlled by younger members of our inner family system who are trying to keep us safe.

Steps to Manage Emotions & Old Beliefs

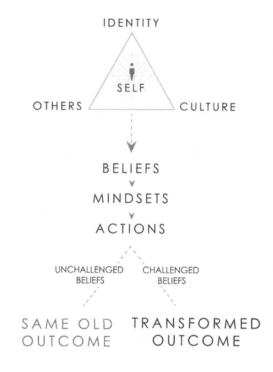

Figure 3. The steps required to challenge old beliefs in order to get to the next level of the journey to transformation.

Below the triangle are three important words: **Beliefs**, **Mindsets** and **Actions**. All prior interactions and experiences create and shape our *Beliefs* about who we are, where we belong, and what we deserve. Based on our beliefs we then develop *Mindsets* or fixed ideas about the way that things are or ought to be, what we tell ourselves, and what we can and cannot do. This has significant effects on the *Actions* we take, which tend to reinforce our mindsets and beliefs and maintain our current identity. Our beliefs and mindsets can prevent us from growing as we get older. They can prevent us from succeeding at tasks we wish to accomplish, reaching goals we set, or letting go of behaviors that don't serve us and that we no longer want. We keep sabotaging our efforts to transform because making changes challenges setpoints created by the triad of our current identity, beliefs, and mindset.

Ancestrally, we are safer if we stay with what is known and continue to get approval from the system. While this may be safe, it limits our potential as humans. We need to stop and evaluate why we do what we do. Unchallenged beliefs lead to the same old outcomes, while challenged beliefs lead to new outcomes. We need to be curious about why we don't succeed at things we are trying to achieve or why our emotions and actions continue to sabotage us.

Most people I know, including myself, my family, and most of my patients, are seeking sustainable change. Sustainable change in any area of our lives requires that we evolve at the level of our identity and beliefs and release patterns of thought and action that no longer serve us.

The way to change, empowerment, and well-being, is to implement The Transformation Steps (Chapter 1) and to take the required steps, as shown here, to challenge old ways of thinking and create new ones.

The next patient's story reveals her journey to achieve lasting change, and how gaining new awareness enabled her to let go of unhealthy habits. We will see how her earlier traumatic experiences created internal family members that tried to protect her but, ultimately, sabotaged her efforts to lose weight. We will also see the importance of changing negative self-talk when we encounter obstacles on the journey towards achieving our goals. We will discover how curiosity and compassion increase awareness and give language to what we are actually feeling, help us challenge old beliefs, restore wholeness in ourselves, and amplify our ability to reach our goals.

Case Study: Teresa's Story

Teresa is a 48-year-old woman who is a nurse, has a diagnosis of obesity, and has a complex medical history. She acquired endocrine deficiencies early in her life, which required the replacement of multiple hormones beginning in early adulthood. She was referred to me by a colleague who knew that I practice mind-body work.

When I met Teresa, she complained that she could not sleep and, despite many efforts, she could not lose weight. Initially, I assumed that her challenges were strictly biological; I figured that the prior treatment for her early endocrine deficiencies may have impacted brain centers that regulate sleep and appetite.

As I interviewed her further, I realized that she had been able to lose weight before. Each time, however, she sabotaged herself and returned to her previous weight. She confided that she started with her best intentions each time; she'd eat well, she'd sleep well, and then something would happen, and she would be back to eating unhealthy foods and drinking three sugary sodas a day.

I was curious: What was that "something" that happened to set her back? "What was going on in your head then?" I asked.

"I do this over and over again. I am bad. I don't seem to follow through. I can't be trusted," she replied.

"Teresa, you know, these comments are not very helpful. If I were saying this to myself and hearing this, I'd actually feel bad. Don't they make you feel bad?" I asked.

"Yeah, they make me feel terrible," she said, lowering her head.

"OK, can we try to be kinder and perhaps less judgmental about what actually happened, so that maybe we can find out what this is really about?"

I provided this response to Teresa because her self-deprecating comments were a distraction to the discussion and an impediment to her growth. I knew it was important to bring my professional, wise-adult self to connect with her without judgment and explore further with her.

"What are you actually feeling?" I asked with compassion and curiosity.

She started to cry. Her vulnerability touched my heart. "Actually," she said, "it's fear. When I was younger, everyone I knew who lost weight in my family died or developed dementia. I don't want to be like my mother. She also lost weight and has dementia. She is counting on me to take care of her now."

"A part of you believes that if you lose weight, you're going to harm yourself and you won't be available to your mother?" I asked, sensing the deep quandary.

"Yes."

"Well, you know that makes sense, given your childhood experiences. I'm sorry you had those losses early in your life. I can see how a younger part of you associated your personal weight loss with losing those you loved."

Even though Teresa was an adult, an educated nurse, and logically understood why and how to lose weight, childhood fears sabotaged her efforts as an adult. Once we translated the feelings of that child-part in her internal family system into language, we understood that she was simply trying to protect herself in a primitive way. By acknowledging the fears of that younger part of herself with compassion, Teresa deepened her awareness and stepped more fully into her innate, wise-adult self. She understood why, up to now, she had been sabotaging her effort at weight loss. She recognized that the younger part of herself had been preventing weight loss to protect herself from the fear of dying. This was part of what had kept the cycle of failure going for so long. By enabling Teresa's wise-adult self to come out and be in charge, Teresa could embrace that child part of her internal family system and reassure her that she was safe. As a wise mother, Teresa explained to her inner child that losing weight would not cause death. Teresa could now be open to a new possibility around weight loss. She noted, as our session ended, "You know, if I ate better, I probably would have more energy. I would be in a better place and more able to take care of my mom."

"Can you think of some ideas of how you can start now to help yourself?" I asked.

She brainstormed some actionable steps she could take before our next appointment and left empowered with new awareness. She had a deeper understanding of the adaptations that her earlier child-mind took on and realized, as a wise-adult, she could handle setbacks differently in the future. As her wise-adult self, Teresa would apply the virtues of curiosity, gratitude, and compassion to her weight-loss journey.

I hope you embrace the power of leaning towards disenfranchised parts of the inner family system with curiosity and compassion. Curiosity and compassion towards our inner child lead to new awareness. When we transform the old stories that have confined us and create new interpretations, meanings, and understandings, we can reach our goals.

My Loving-Kindness Wish for You

May you be curious
May you listen
May you embrace your inner children
May you be whole

Meditation to Enhance Your Journaling

Please scan the QR Code with your Smartphone or follow this link: https://youtu.be/gkyEtt-8piU

Journaling for Transformation

I invite you to look at the area in your life that you're trying to improve. To enhance your reflection, I have provided a list of questions to support you as you consider what may be holding you back.

1. Envision the area of your life that you want to improve. Without judgment, ask yourself the following questions and reflect with curiosity and compassion:
   - What is it that you really yearn for?
   - What is blocking or getting in the way of your progress?
   - What happens when you try to move forward?
   - Why is it that you're not getting to do what you want?
   - What do you do or not do? Is there a pattern?

- Do you procrastinate? Do you miss appointments with yourself? Do you check out?
- Is your inner critic saying unkind things, listing why you don't deserve to have what you want, filling you with guilt and shame? If so, lovingly release this part of yourself. Let your wiser, more mature self, take charge.

Be patient. When you hear an answer from that younger part of you, listen with empathy. Then validate and accept what it is as it is.

2. With compassion, proceed to ask the next set of questions and practice curiosity.

- What beliefs do you have about yourself and others?
- What might happen if you were to successfully change in this area of your life?
- Do you have fears of succeeding? Why? Do you have any fears of intimacy? What might this be about? Do you fear for your safety? Explain.
- Do you have fears of loss? How so?
- What do you fear remembering? How can you become more compassionate and loving of yourself despite these difficult memories and past experiences?
- Is it possible that these beliefs that you have from an older time may not be true now?
- Where in your body does this sadness or frustration from the past live?
- Can you send love and attention to that part of your body?
- Is there a part of you that feels that you don't deserve to receive the outcomes of your desires?
- How else can you think about this now?

Now, return to the energetic bond of your heart's intelligence and your wise and highest essence and send empathy and loving support. Hold that part of you that has been vulnerable, that has suffered and exerted so much energy trying to protect you. Let that part of you, that inner child, know that you honor their perspective. Thank the inner child for all it has done to try to help you. Lovingly inform this part of you that it can trust the wise-adult guide that is now there.

Allow yourself to consciously rest. Take in a few more breaths. Fully embody this beautiful integration. Every part of you is good. Every part of you is worthy and deserving of having what you want. Fully sense the gifts that come from being receptive to ourselves and living in the questions.

Chapter 3

Emotions, Habits & Stress

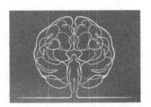

The Secret Language of Mind-Body Interactions

All of us experience emotions, and most of us know that the stresses of life impact our emotional well-being. But perhaps we are not as aware of the degree that stress and emotions can influence the health of the body. In this part of the "care of our mind" journey, we will develop an understanding of how our emotions affect our body and mind and how our mind and body react to them. When the mind reacts to emotions, our biology shifts toward a hard-wired, ancestrally-evolved flight-fight response. If we chronically react, we age faster and become exhausted. How can we learn to shift from triggered patterns of reacting that make us ill to more empowered responses?

When we learn to identify our emotions and their triggers, we can mindfully respond rather than react to them. We can be more conscious about the sources of our stress so we can limit them. We have choices. Do we continue to ignore and numb our emotions and succumb to stress, or do we lean in with curiosity to try and understand what they are communicating and doing to us?

We can counteract the ever-present impact and negative effects of stress. With new awareness, we *can* develop the capacity of curiosity and listen to what our emotions have to say to us. And we can manifest our desires by revising old, disempowered interpretations of these emotions into new and empowered meanings.

My Story

Let me tell you a story from my early doctor days to bring to life the concept of mind-body interplay and our ancestral stress-responsive survival system. When I was a chief resident, I was given the opportunity to present at Grand Rounds, a weekly meeting that doctors and students attend to hear about and discuss new science and medical cases. If a medical case is presented, the evaluation of the patient, the thought processes behind the care, and potential treatment options are discussed. In most teaching hospitals, this kind of presentation happens in a big auditorium with 50 to 100 doctors and students attending.

I stood on the stage behind the podium prepared to start my slide presentation. A part of me felt prepared to present. I knew my stuff. I wanted to do a good job. Another part of me was filled with *dread*. I felt tightness in my throat. I looked out at all of the doctors and students. As the lights dimmed, I began to see flashes in my eyes. Sweat drenched my body, the room swirled around me, and everything went black. I passed out. I regained consciousness on the floor. The doctors were slowly departing the auditorium. Nobody came up to the stage to help me. Perhaps, like me, they were horrified by what they were seeing. Perhaps they saw in me their younger, less-assured selves.

As I reflected on this situation, I realized that an inner, younger part of me felt highly insecure. This younger part of me was not sure that I had a *perfect* understanding of what I was presenting and wrestled with believing that I belonged in that space. She felt like an impostor—not an unusual inner experience for young doctors and other professionals. When I went up on the stage, I was unaware that this emotional drama was taking place in my mind; deep inside, a part of me felt like I wasn't *enough* to do this presentation. Being unaware, all I sensed was that I was physically unwell and then found myself on the floor.

My story is an example of a mind-body interaction. My inner emotions (fear of failure and perfectionism) and beliefs (I am not ready, I'm not good enough, I don't belong here) led to a strong physical reaction from my autonomic nervous system. The less mature part of me believed that I was not a capable enough doctor to present material to other doctors. These beliefs impacted my actual physiology and reduced my blood pressure enough that I literally checked out by passing out. Then, the embarrassment and humiliation I felt upon watching all the doctors leave the auditorium, along with my inability to present the case, served to further confirm the inner belief that I was not a good enough or capable enough doctor. Fortunately, I've come a long way since then. Now, I love making and offering presentations and see them as opportunities to serve others by sharing valuable information.

Emotions, Stress & the Nervous System

Various factors—our beliefs, ideas, health, mindset, choices, behaviors, etc.—determine the quality of our lives. Emotions also influence our well-being. Most of us think of emotions as strong feelings or moods towards people, places, activities or things in our environment. These emotions can drive our behavior. What's often not discussed is the actual biology, or physiology, of emotions. Biologically, emotions are a network of nerve cells that fire together and send out chemical signals when stimulated by scents, events, places, memories, and people. Emotions change the chemistry of our cells in both the body and the brain.

So, what about stress, which is pervasive in our day-to-day lives? Stress is any change contributing to physical, emotional, or mental pressures. Stress destabilizes us from the body-mind's central homeostatic or stable balanced state. Stress is a normal part of life and can be good and bad for us. It can be positive, such as when we are exercising or when we are preparing for a performance in which we hope to excel. These good responses to stress can build resilience, grit, and physical and mental strength. On the other hand, stress regularly perceived as threatening our survival, such as in childhood trauma or post-traumatic stress disorder (PTSD), is harmful. This type of stress triggers and overwhelms the sympathetic nervous system to continually experience fight-flight-freeze mode.

In order to fully appreciate triggered body reactions, we must understand that there are two divisions of the autonomic nervous system: the parasympathetic and sympathetic nervous systems. The parasympathetic nervous system brings the body back to a calm state after stress and overworking. This is our 10th cranial nerve, the vagus nerve. This nerve uses acetylcholine as its neurotransmitter and has varied functions in the body. The vagus nerve handles all involuntary processes such as heart rate, blood pressure, respiration, and digestion. This neurotransmitter calms us after stressful events and brings us back to stability.

Loss of consciousness is a function of the vagus nerve that is rarely discussed but not infrequently experienced. This may occur after unexpected or severe pain and emotions. I experienced this when I passed out during Grand Rounds. Both my blood pressure and heart rate dropped. Less blood went to my brain, causing lightheadedness, flashing lights, and ultimately causing me to pass out. By lying down, I improved brain blood flow and reconnected to my senses. Loss of consciousness is what we medically refer to as a *vasovagal* response. When this third branch of the vagus is activated by severe emotional stress, as I experienced, it disconnects one from experiencing what is happening. It disconnects the mind from the body and its sensations.

While the parasympathetic nervous system or the vagus nerve calms us during stress, the sympathetic nervous system has a different function. The sympathetic nervous system remains on sensory alert for potential danger in the environment and prepares the body for fight-flight-freeze responses. These fight-flight-freeze responses are often referred to as ancestral stress responses. We contract. We fight by discharging our power physically or verbally. We flee by checking out physically or emotionally. We freeze by becoming immobilized or disconnected.

Some of these ancestral responses are life-saving in the appropriate setting and some no longer serve us and may lead to habits that cause psychological pain, disenfranchisement and negative mind-body outcomes.

What Happens to Our Mind and Body When We Are Stressed?

When we are triggered by stress or difficult emotions, our whole body is ignited with the sensation to fight or to run from the inciting person or event—or the *tiger*. This sensation is so overpowering we don't even feel pain. If we're able to fight off, run away from, or avoid the oppressor—or *tiger*—that caused the stress, we can relax and return to equilibrium. But if the stress is ongoing, then the fight-flight-freeze system remains on, especially if we have little to no support and resources to effectively deal with these stressful situations.

And stressful situations abound. Some of us may feel stuck in a bad job situation with no flexibility, or an economic crisis with mounting fears of not meeting the bills, or ongoing conflict or abuse in a personal or professional relationship, or loneliness, or grief. There is no shortage to stress, no shortage to the effects on our mind and also our body.

When the fight-flight-freeze system is triggered, different chemical signals are sent throughout the body to prepare for the challenge. Cortisol and adrenaline are secreted from the adrenal glands. Our heart rate increases and is less variable. Our blood vessels tighten and blood pressure increases, and our glucose levels go up. Our gut does not work as effectively, and we may experience constipation, diarrhea, indigestion, reflux, or irritable bowel syndrome. This is because the vagus or calming nerve is less functional when we are stressed and the sympathetic, or fight-flight-freeze system, is on. If this goes on for extended periods of time, muscle tension increases and we feel as if we have the flu, our energy levels decrease, and exhaustion overtakes us. We struggle to sleep because stress makes us hypervigilant. Our moods change. We feel irritable, anxious, and depressed. Our threshold to become irritable is lowered. We *react* to things rather than *respond* wisely. Our body is inflamed. Our immunity decreases, and we catch every flu and virus going around. The calorie-burning rate slows down and we are hungrier, so we gain weight. Sex hormones are lowered, and along with that, your sex drive. The telomeres, or protective end caps of chromosomes, shorten, which causes premature aging and increases our mortality rates.

Stress-related conditions are the most common reasons that patients go to doctors. Many of us suffer from depression and anxiety. These mood states may be situational, familial, or seasonal in origin. In all cases, during these times we have a shift or chemical imbalance that is different from when we are not in those states. Recent research explores the limitations of cognition to manage the negative emotions from the stress that we increasingly experience. This research also examines the imbalance between an overactive sympathetic nervous system and an underactive vagus-related calming response.

The more we understand our nervous system, emotions, the impact of stress and how to consciously handle those moments when we are triggered, the more we can create positive outcomes in our personal and professional relationships. *We can help ourselves.* We can develop skills to deal effectively with our emotions. We can learn to interpret everyday stress and crises more favorably. We can learn to calm our nervous system by knowing how to increase the activity of our vagus nerve—or calming nerve. We can create peace in the midst of chaos and thereby enhance our overall health and wellness.

Transform Patterned Reactions to Empowered Responses

If we are not consciously aware of the meanings we make of our emotions or feelings, then we *allow* our more primitive interpretations and subsequent responses and habits to happen unchallenged. I invite you to take charge of your emotions. I've created two visual models to illustrate old ways and new possibilities of responding when we are triggered (Figures 3 and 4). I've also provided a QR code to a guided meditation that will center and calm you before you try to work with emotions. Please do this work in a safe place and remember this work is an adjunct but does not replace ongoing psychiatric care. These models will support you in developing the skills of managing your emotions and feelings so that your most empowered self can be in charge rather than your emotions. Let's examine these two charts in detail.

Figure 4 is a model illustration to enhance our awareness of what typically happens when we are triggered and feelings, emotional reactions, and behaviors are activated.

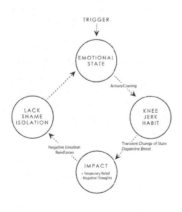

Triggers & Habits

Copyright © Dr. Beatriz Olson 2023

Figure 4. Soothing-based actions and negative self-talk triggered by an emotional state. This is also the cycle of how a habit can be formed and maintained.

47

Note the four circles connected by four arrows that travel in a clockwise direction. These circles illustrate the typical process of unconscious ancestral-patterned reactions to stress: we are triggered by something that activates an emotional state. Emotions cause us to take action or do something to change how we feel. This is when we crave the things that provide temporary relief or distract us from what has occurred. Eating a tub of ice cream, drinking too much, surfing the net for hours—these serve the craving through providing a dopamine (positive energy) boost. This boost temporarily calms us down and distracts us from what is happening. Shortly after we serve the craving and do something unhealthy, we feel bad because the behaviors were not aligned with our goals or serving who we really are. We may criticize or shame ourselves, thinking this will help, but derogatory comments never help, nor do they change behaviors, whether your own or someone else's. It only reinforces our negative emotions, lack of control, increased shame and keeps us isolated from others. This sustains a state of non-possibility. If our old feelings, behaviors, and reactions remain unchallenged, the cycle begins again with the next trigger. In these cycles, a soothing behavior, repeated enough, can become a habit. These habits continue even if we don't like them and want to change them.

Figure 5 provides a more conscious, thoughtful, and empowered way to respond to stress. Take a short 2-minute timeout to breathe and connect to yourself. Ask yourself three questions to ask the angsty and craving mind:

1) Why are you really craving the particular food/action/thing now?
2) What are you actually feeling?
3) Where are you feeling or sensing this anxiety in the body?

Exploring these three questions creates a space for reassessing the action that was ultimately not going to help you. This short skill-developing practice will empower you to take more life-affirming actions. You will begin to replace old habits and actions you have wanted to change. By challenging your old ways of being, you naturally transform and evolve your responses from old thoughts, beliefs, and emotions to new and empowered ones. Developing such skills can serve us all to create happier and more connected relationships at home, work, and life.

Nurturing Ways to Transform
Old into New Habits

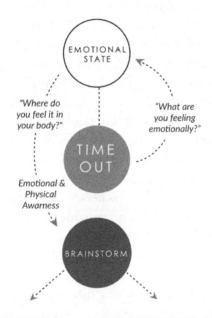

Figure 5. Nurturing ways to transform old habits and behaviors into new ones that are aligned with our values and well-healthy goals.

Recently, the Russian invasion of Ukraine caused extreme angst for me. This led me to eat cheddar cheese and crackers (which I never do) as I watched the evening news. The crunch and salty fat sensory experience soothed me. I rarely snack after dinner and did not like this new behavior. I initially felt badly about myself for doing something I normally don't do and coach others not to do.

The angsty-anxious physical feeling and the new cracker and cheese night-eating behavior made me curious. Why was I feeling so angsty? Why was I engaging in emotional eating? I took a "mindful timeout" to meditate and reflect. I asked myself, "what are you really feeling?" I realized that the invasion of Ukraine reminded the 5- to 6-year-old younger part of me of the suffering, fear, and lack of control and choice that my family had while living in communist Cuba. This younger part felt immense fear of harm that could come to her family and sadness that she could not help. No one could help. Once I understood this, I was able, as my wise-adult self, to embrace this young and worried inner family member. I became a compassionate witness to her suffering and efforts to make "us" feel better by eating the salty crackers. The combination of taking a timeout to meditate, reflect and provide compassion to a younger part of myself resulted in the end of post-dinner snacking to calm my emotions.

Being curious about our emotions disrupts knee-jerk reactivity to old mindsets and habitual responses to stress. Being compassionate with ourselves is transformative. This is the antidote to our useless derogatory, perfectionistic and abusive self-dialogue. As you can see from Figure 5, remaining attuned to our emotional states is important. When we notice that we are struggling with more difficult emotional states, we must learn to pause and take a healthy timeout. During this timeout, we reflect on what we are feeling and where we feel the emotions in our body. Rather than react in the same old ways, we take time to brainstorm on new possibilities, new options, and new choices that our new and empowered self can make instead.

Similarly, the story I shared earlier about fainting before an important presentation to doctors, revealed my own sense of inadequacy and my body's strong reaction to pull me out of the event. I learned to transform my shame and perfectionism into a more compassionate relationship with myself. I turned my fear of failure and rejection into curiosity. I have learned to take a timeout and ask myself, "What is really happening here? What are my actual thoughts about this situation? How can I see this differently?" Bringing to awareness my reflections on the situation was how I learned to understand the secret language and stories held by my mind's emotions. When we open our minds and listen with compassion to what is being thought and felt by our younger-inner parts, we can see that the younger parts of us are reacting to old triggers and displaying primitive responses. Learning to label our emotions accurately and translate into words our body-mind experiences enable us to understand our responses and behaviors. This process best happens without judging ourselves. It is a compassionate inquiry. We can embrace the younger and often more wounded parts of ourselves. We begin shifting our primitive interpretations from a less conscious awareness to a more enlightened interpretation from a higher level of conscious awareness. The new meanings that emerge improve the quality of our perspectives, decrease suffering, and empower ourselves. The process illustrated in Figure 5 supports us to integrate disenfranchised younger parts of ourselves into our wholeness.

Remember, we are all human. We experience stress, distorted types of thinking and cope in a variety of ways that are not productive. We can curb the tendencies to act out by developing the virtues of curiosity and compassion. We can explore our younger self and discover new meanings to our emotions. These are the skills required to manage stress and emotions in a more mature and healthy way.

Additional Stress Reduction Techniques

Most people are unaware that we can access the calming nervous system on demand and that this can be lifesaving. Our capacity to activate our own relaxation response was popularized in the '70s by Herbert Benson of Harvard University. He demystified the concept of meditation and taught that anyone could calm their nervous system by focusing on breathing, without expensive mantras or religiosity. He found that meditation is simply a way to stimulate the vagus nerve, our good old calming parasympathetic system. We can achieve a sense of calm by taking slow, deep breaths, with or without the repetition of words, phrases, mantras, or heart-mind focused metta—positive intentions or prayer for wellness for oneself or others. Benson demonstrated that meditation led to a decrease in blood pressure and heart disease in general. Meditation created a sense of well-being for participants.

Later, Jon Kabat-Zinn popularized the concept of mindfulness-based meditation and stress reduction by using breath and present moment awareness. He emphasized the importance of being in the here and now. Whether one meditated with or without movement, he taught that being present or mindful of our breath enhanced wellness and decreased the perception of stress, pain, and suffering. Additionally, mindfulness-based meditation has been shown to decrease depression and anxiety, improve sleep, lower blood pressure and pulse rate, and decrease anxiety prior to medical procedures. Finally, mindfulness-based stress reduction studies show that people who meditate have growing empathy and compassion for themselves and others. Compared to non-meditators, meditators perform as if they were seven years younger when doing complex mental tasks and memory tests.

Stress reduction techniques can interrupt and change old ways of dealing with emotions, stress, and established patterns of logic, mindsets, and behavior. Using techniques like meditation enable us to perceive our life with a more nurturing perspective. There is no shortage of stress-reducing modalities. Some of us may prefer moving meditations (breath and movement), like yoga, Tai Chi, or Qigong. Others may prefer body scanning—lying down or sitting and scanning different parts of our body to sense where there is tension and where there is not. There are numerous ways to connect to our body, mind, higher consciousness, and spirit in order to calm ourselves when stressed.

My Go-To Meditation Method

For the past 25 years, a regular meditation practice has transformed me into a calmer and more compassionate human, despite the limitations and effects of childhood and adult trauma. I've benefited from learning meditation techniques with Deepak Chopra and David Simon who were teaching together in La Jolla, California and Goa, India, in the 1990s. Shortly after, I also engaged in mindfulness training from my Buddhist colleague Seth Zuihō Segall, who learned from Jon Kabat-Zinn. Though I've practiced numerous techniques, I find the simplest and most effective method is to connect to the breath cycle. Breath gives us life and energy. Oxygen calms down the nervous system.

The way I personally engage in breathwork is to find a comfortable place. Then I focus on sensing my buttocks on the surface of my chair to become more aware of my body. I breathe in through my nose and feel the sensation of air entering through my nose. My in-breath fills my lungs and expands my abdomen. Connected to my seat and to my breath, I continue. I count silently to four as I inhale and count silently to six as I exhale. A slightly longer out-breath followed by a pause before I take the next in-breath is deeply calming to the nervous system and the mind-body unit. Sometimes, when I reach the pause between the in- and out-breath, I silently state a word, or mantra, like peace, calm, love or om. Some people may prefer to say "in" when they are breathing in and "out" when they are breathing out.

Taking two to five minutes to breathe reboots our inner nervous operating system. These brief periods of breathing, as quick as a bathroom break, can enhance our focus and learning abilities. I have taught this technique to anxious or panicky patients, to students in my online courses, and to doctors during my self-care lectures. Check out the many guided mind-body calming and aligning meditations recommended at the end of each chapter and in the resource section at the end of the book.

Meditation and mindfulness are *practices*. Sometimes new practitioners feel discouraged when they notice they are thinking a lot of thoughts rather than meditating. The normal function of the mind, however, is to think. Even seasoned meditators notice thoughts. When this happens, stop engaging with the thought, say goodbye to it, and go back to focusing on the breath. After some time, one learns that thoughts come and go. We can observe them without paying attention to or engaging with them. We can also label thoughts as *neutral* or *judgmental* before we let them float off. With time, curiosity, and dedication to our practice, we start to experience more spaciousness and less attachment to our thoughts. The quality of our thoughts improves. We start to notice that we are responding more consciously rather than reacting to whatever is happening inside and around us. Emotions and the actions of others no longer control us.

Trauma and the Freeze Stress Response

Trauma is an emotional response to extreme events that cause short and long-term reactions. Most of us will experience some kind of traumatic event in our lives. At the time of such events, we can't logically register and express or give language to what is happening. We can't create a coherent story. We may feel overwhelming fear and a huge sense of loss and helplessness. We also may experience physical symptoms like headaches or gastrointestinal problems. The result is the establishment of post-traumatic neural pathways.

When any stimulus reminiscent of the initial trauma triggers these pathways, traumatized individuals vividly re-experience the same emotional and physical response and suffering they did during the original experience. We may be unable or incapable of leaving the unpleasant or unwanted event, person, or place we are facing and experience continual trauma and oppression. When this happens, a part of the autonomic nervous system kicks in to defend us. We may "freeze" and stop feeling; we checkout.

Such is the case with many veterans, survivors of bombings, survivors of school gun violence or childhood trauma. Their experiences were unexpected, painful, and unavoidable. The result is that many trauma survivors resort to alcohol or drugs to distract themselves from reliving their trauma. Special healing techniques and help from trauma experts are required to decrease this type of repetitive suffering.

Healing for trauma victims is complex. It requires working with the mind *and* the body since the body holds the 'horror experiences' in its sinews. If you are a victim or know someone who has endured trauma, I invite you to read Bessel van der Kolk's book *The Body Keeps the Score* and Donald Kalsched's *The Inner World of Trauma*.

Another resource is to find a therapist that practices Eye Movement Desensitization and Reprocessing (EMDR). Such a therapist will guide a patient through this evidence-based technique. The patient will briefly share the story of their trauma while simultaneously moving their eyes back and forth to experience bilateral stimulation. This technique allows the story to get passively transferred through the corpus callosum (the area connecting the two sides of the brain) to the brain's more intellectual side. This enables the emotions and story to become more integrated in real time and space in the brain, allowing for less suffering and physical reactivity when emotions associated with the traumatic event are triggered. Combining these techniques with physical work like yoga and movement help to process and remove the pain from where it has been stored in the body. These techniques can let traumatized people feel, at some point, whole again.

Change Begins Now

Learning to cultivate stress-reduction skills gives you the ability to shift the balance from the activated sympathetic, or flight-fight-freeze response, to a more peaceful space. The meditative techniques described in this chapter connect and align the mind to the body. When the body and mind are calmed and aligned, you can access the higher centers of your brain with conscious creativity, imagination, and connection to a personal and shared spiritual nature.

My Loving-Kindness Wish for You

May you have peace and joy in your life
May you find your method to calm your mind and body
May you be wisely responsive, flexible, and creative.

Meditation to Enhance Your Journaling

Please scan the QR Code with your Smartphone or follow this link: https://youtu.be/wZ4CefYgkG8

Journaling for Transformation

Managing Emotions and Habitual Reactions

To review, when we are triggered into complex emotional states, we need to take a "timeout" and stop before we act. During this timeout, we focus on being curious and compassionate. This is the way to uncover the meaning that we are making of the feelings and emotions.

1. The following are some questions we can ask ourselves when we don't feel quite right or experience angst. If we lean in, listen and explore the journal questions below, we will uncover new insights to what is really going on with ourselves.

   - Why do I need to do this now?
   - What was I just thinking or feeling before this started?
   - What part of me is thinking it must satisfy a craving or engage in numbing behavior?
   - How old is this part of me?
   - What is the real issue here? What happened? What were the circumstances?
   - What am I actually feeling (sad, anxious, angry, scared, lonely)?
   - What are the beliefs that have been associated with this emotion?
   - Where in the body is this feeling located?
   - What is the sensation of this in my body?
   - (tightness in my throat, my chest, stomach, nausea.)
   - What is it that I really need or want now?
   - Does this thinking or emotion make sense now?
   - How can I look at this situation differently?
   - What else can I do that will soothe me or my distressed inner family member(s)?
   - How can I more effectively support my current values and interests?

Together, our wise-adult self and our inner child can explore and reinterpret the old thinking to create new meanings and ways to respond and behave when the same emotion is triggered in the future. Like all things, this process takes practice, and with practice comes transformation.

2. I invite you to consider the following questions, as these will give you insights into areas that you might want to improve to develop a better and more compassionate relationship with yourself:

    • What do you do when things don't go your way? When you are disappointed? When you do not feel right?
    • Do you blame yourself? Do you blame others? How so?
    • What meaning do you make of difficult situations?
    • How have you been hurt or victimized? What do you feel about being hurt? How can you create new meanings from these situations that empower you?
    • Do you take time to reflect upon difficult and disappointing circumstances?
    • How can you get support and improve the situation?
    • What do you do to calm yourself? Does this help you and for how long?
    • How can you remind yourself that cravings are short-lasting and temporary and will not resolve the stress and emotions that caused them?

Letting go of the old and familiar ways of handling physical and mental stress, fatigue, and disappointments involves evaluating your triggers, thoughts, emotions, old beliefs, and actions. Our patterns may feel familiar and comfortable, but these patterns keep us locked in contraction and prevent our growth and possibility for change.

Managing Stress

Something all of us do, especially women, is multitasking. Multitasking stresses the brain and body. Notice that when you are trying to do more than one activity at a time, this stresses your body. Reflect on how you can reduce the patterns of multitasking.

Take some time to consider and evaluate stress in your life in the following domains below.

3. Ask yourself how you can go about improving the situation in these various areas of your life. Lean in with curiosity. What causes stress or suffering in these areas? What can you do? Be creative? Can you shift things around to have more quality time with yourself and those you love? Can you add more goodness to your schedule? Who can you ask to support you? What do you need to say to make things better?

- Home
- Work
- Partner/spouse
- Family member (child/parent/pet)
- You
- Environment
- Government
- News
- World/climate
- Worry/anxiety/depression
- Finances
- Your safety
- Your health

4. Consider the following ways to better manage stress and dissatisfaction. Which ones below can you try?

- Take a mindful moment to sit, breathe and center your body.
- Lie down and close your eyes for 15 minutes listening to something you like.
- Hang out with someone who unconditionally loves you like your pet or your young child.
- Exercise, move, stretch, do yoga moves (these all increase telomeres!).
- Call a friend, talk it out.
- Drink tea.

- Listen to music.
- Watch TV or social media that makes you laugh.
- Do a hobby, do some artwork, or work on a project.
- Clean and declutter
- Find and take an online meditation or yoga class.
- Rest
- Establish healthy sleep habits.

Care of The Body

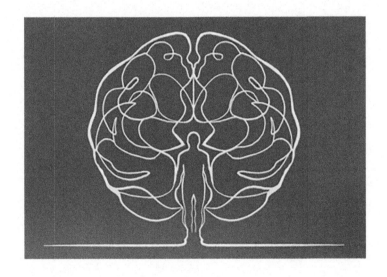

Chapter 4

What to Eat, When & Why

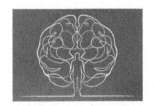

Food as Medicine

How did our ancestral metabolism system evolve over thousands of years enabling us to survive when food scarcity was the norm? How do we overcome our ancestral wiring now that food abundance is the norm? Reflecting on these questions and understanding how our body and brain interprets and metabolizes the foods we eat can support us in our efforts to increase our energy and attain a healthier body and weight. Broader knowledge of the ancestral metabolism system and nutrition is necessary to help us address the obesity and diabetes epidemics we are currently facing, and their impact on future generations.

I teach my patients how nutrient-dense whole foods are our best medicine. Such foods provide information for the body and brain. Choosing the foods that our body needs, instead of what it craves, is a key concept to learn. I encourage my patients to develop curiosity about their mindset and old-conditioned thoughts about when, what and how much to eat. I share my experiences around not giving in to cravings. Cravings have biological and emotional origins. Discerning the source of where our cravings come from and the biology that drives them is empowering.

Over the years, I have gathered information about the complex metabolism of nutrients and have used this information to alter how and when I eat. This awareness guides my choices; I have learned to say 'no' to my ancestral survival-driven food cravings. Additionally, I regulated my dysfunctional metabolism and weight by using food as medicine and allowing my digestive system and liver to work optimally for me. With these changes, I feel energetic and have sustained a healthy weight for decades.

My Story

When I went to medical school, I understood that we eat to receive energy, we breathe to live, and we drink water to keep hydrated. However, the details of how all this happened were unclear to me. Up to that time, I believed that I was eating the right foods at the right time, based on how I saw others eat and what was advertised on TV. As new immigrants to America, my family had limited money and mostly bought processed foods because they were cheaper. On Sundays, it was a luxury for my mother and me not to cook at home. Our big family adventure was to go to White Castle, Burger King or McDonald's and enjoy cheeseburgers, fries, and ice cream shakes. Back then, we didn't understand that lesser amounts of high-quality, nutrient-dense foods would have been better for our health.

At that time, my mother and I cooked dinners at home, which consisted of whole foods, like plantains, beans, rice, meats and salad (iceberg lettuce). Even with all these food options, I was hungrier than I had been in the past. I craved and ate unhealthy foods like Entenmann's sweet rolls and waffles with butter and maple syrup for breakfast. I craved snacks such as Twinkies, saltine crackers with cream cheese and orange marmalade, and big glasses of milk. And I gained weight. Curiously, the rest of my family did not appear to be so hungry and did not gain weight. For a few months, I tried bulimia as a method to lose weight, but it did not diminish my hunger, my weight, or self-dissatisfaction.

Thankfully, I've learned a lot about why I had such rapid weight gain at that time in my life, how the body interprets the foods we eat, and fights to keep our highest weight. More importantly, I've learned how to help others prevent disordered eating and weight gain or regain.

The Ancestral Brain & Food Cravings

Thousands of years ago, our bodies and minds adapted to survive food scarcity. During these periods of scarcity, the body utilized its energy fat stores and broke down old cells that were no longer working well to keep us healthy. When food was available, the body maintained and supported weight gain. The ancestral brain is genetically encoded to seek sweet-tasting foods and store such foods in the body when they are available. Despite the abundance of sugar-rich foods today, these old evolutionary adaptations continue to cause us to crave and eat sweet foods and gain excess weight, even if we seek neither. Satisfying these cravings gives the ancestral mind pleasure and security. The genetic encoding to seek food, especially sweets, accomplishes two things: it increases our likelihood of surviving famine and passes these protective instincts on to our children.

Energy Produced by Our Cell's Mitochondria

Our cells are precious and require special loving care. They work day and night, tending to the needs of the body. They protect DNA in the nucleus. They make proteins needed from DNA messages. They eliminate toxicities that accumulate after a cell's day of hard work. Cells make energy in the fabulous *mitochondria* so the body will work and feel well. The mitochondria, beautiful little bean-shaped organelles, live inside every cell in the body and are crucial for the functioning of our body. They transform food into energy for our body to live. Mitochondria create our energy using three sources:

1. **Food:** Mitochondria transform food into energy by converting glucose, amino acids, and fatty acids into energy. Glucose is the primary form of carbohydrates/

sugars in the blood. Amino acids are molecules that form proteins. Fatty acids are the building blocks of fat in our bodies and in our food.

2. **Water:** Water makes up about 70 percent of our body and is necessary to support the structure and functioning of our cells. Water is an essential component for cells to make energy. A loss of 4 percent of water leads to dehydration, and a loss of 15 percent can lead to death. Since we lose water due to respiration, sweat, and waste, we must replace this loss by consuming water in the form of liquids, fruits, and vegetables.

3. **Oxygen:** Mitochondria use oxygen to make and provide the energy needed to survive. Oxygen provides our cells with the energy to break down food. Oxygen gets into the cells from the air that we breathe into our lungs. Red blood cells transport oxygen from our lungs into our blood vessels throughout the whole body.

Another important term to know is *Adenosine Triphosphate* or ATP. ATP is a molecule and the predominant energy currency that all living cells use to do their work. ATP enables all cells, organs like the brain, and other systems in the body to function. Without this energy currency, the muscles, including our heart, cannot work. If food, water, or air are lacking or unable to get to where they need to for the cell's energy factories, the mitochondria can't make ATP, the body has less energy, and we feel tired.

You may know someone, for example, who, during the early stages of the Covid pandemic, contracted the virus and was hospitalized because they struggled to breathe and required high concentrations of oxygen to survive. Their mitochondria were losing the ability to make energy for them due to the lack of oxygen. They needed our great conventional medicine and highly trained medical professionals to save their lives by providing high concentrations of oxygen to overcome the deficit caused by lung inflammation.

What Damages Mitochondria & Accelerates Aging

When our cell's mitochondria malfunction and become sick, we lose energy and age faster. *Inflammation, oxidative stress, the wrong nutrition and overnutrition, and environmental or lifestyle-related factors* all cause mitochondria to break down faster. A symptom of mitochondrial breakdown is fatigue. We need to be aware of the factors that make mitochondria function poorly because they make us unwell. Then we can do something about protecting them and ourselves from harm. We have a choice about how we care for our mitochondria, how much energy we have, and how rapidly we age.

Signs of inflammation include swelling, pain and tiredness. Inflammation is the body's natural immune response to fight bacterial or viral invaders, irritants, and toxins. During inflammation, immune cells release signaling proteins or cytokines that cause acute damage. In chronic inflammation, this process goes on and on. When chronic inflammation and oxidative stress are not contained, we damage our cells, mitochondria, and DNA. The inflammatory cytokines also make the lining of our blood vessels unstable, making them vulnerable to cholesterol deposits, which increases the risk of heart disease, heart attacks, and stroke. Other chronic inflammatory conditions include autoimmune diseases, fatty liver and hepatitis, diabetes, depression, inflammatory bowel problems including dysbiosis and leaky gut, rheumatoid or psoriatic arthritis, heart disease, and Alzheimer's disease. Inflammation and its related oxidative stress can overwhelm our natural ability to use or produce antioxidants to manage this metabolic havoc. This sabotages the capacity of our cells to recover and function effectively.

Oxidative stress is created by free radicals, which are unstable molecules that damage our cells. Every cell in our body naturally makes these nasty molecules while doing its daily work. These daily oxidative hits can damage both the cell's machinery and DNA. Fortunately, the body has a natural way of protecting the cells from free radicals and neutralizing their damage with antioxidants, glutathione, and vitamins C and E. Our liver helps us further by getting rid of toxic substances, including metabolized hormones and other waste. Like chronic inflammation, chronic oxidative stress can damage the mitochondria, and this causes our cells to age faster and stop working. These aged cells also release their own SOS inflammation signals around them. These senescent or "zombie" cells speed up the aging process in the body and set the stage for the onset of chronic diseases, cancer, and cognitive decline. We can help the body create antioxidants when we consume colorful fruits, vegetables, and citrus. We can help the liver metabolize hormones better by eating more brussel sprouts, broccoli, cabbage, and cauliflower. We can get rid of these senescent cells by allowing our bodies to use them as "food" during periods of fasting.

Lifestyle choices, environmental factors, and viruses also play significant roles in creating chronic inflammation and oxidative stress. Poor nutrition and excess food, not enough sleep, a sedentary lifestyle, inadequate stress management, tobacco use, excessive alcohol use, and too much or too little exercise all increase free radical activity. Air, water, and soil pollution, radiation exposure, and pesticides accelerate cellular aging by creating chronic inflammatory states and oxidative stress. The good news is that many of these factors are under our control. We have a choice about how we live our life and what we allow to happen in our body.

Stress may be physical, psychological, or environmental and contributes to the establishment of an unhealthy metabolic legacy. Stress is inflammatory and causes oxidative stress to our cells. This causes our body and brain to age more rapidly. It causes digestive and immune dysfunction, overactivation of our nervous system, slows down metabolism, increases weight gain and rates of anxiety and depression. Stress-related metabolic dysfunction can be overcome by learning about stress and using stress reduction techniques regularly, as we discussed earlier in the book.

Our access to quality nutrition affects not just our cell's energy production and function but also how we manage our appetite, metabolism, and weight. We live in what scientists call an "obesogenic environment," which means food is *everywhere*. Stress, poor sleep, lack of exercise, and disrespect for our natural body rhythms all increase our struggles with excess weight. Since food is always available, we eat too much and too frequently throughout the day. We regularly choose high-fat, highly processed refined carbohydrates and sugar-sweetened foods. These types of food and high-frequency eating cause metabolic dysfunction, inflammation, and oxidative stress.

I am driven to share information crucial to our survival. Knowledge is power. Knowing about nutrition, metabolism, and the origins of biological cravings, we can *choose* the right foods and lifestyle for our bodies. This knowledge allows us to challenge our responses to ancestral drives and wiring. Knowledge and curiosity enable us to realize that we will not perish by letting ourselves be hungry, allowing longer periods of time between meals (without snacking), and choosing more plant-based whole foods, which make us feel fuller. Long periods of not eating allow the liver and mitochondria to work better and the body to heal itself, eventually returning to a healthy weight and age more slowly. From my experience, it is possible to train the conscious brain to disregard ancestral drives related to hunger, but it takes knowledge to make the best choices and a conscious effort, along with practice.

Nutrition Facts Essential for Good Health

I have been helping patients for years understand that despite what was taught to me in medical school, a calorie is not always a calorie. Calories are a basic description of how much energy is expected from a given nutrient (carbohydrates, proteins and fats). For example, if you eat one gram of lean protein, you get four calories (4 per gram). The same is true for carbohydrates, whether they're simple (sugar, flour, boxed cereals, pasta, bread, rice) or complex (starchy and non-starchy vegetables, fruits, potatoes, etc.); they all have four calories per gram. So, if all the calories you eat were totally absorbed, whether they are 15 grams of carbohydrates or 15 grams of protein, they would provide 60 calories of energy to the body. In comparison, fats deliver the most energy per gram, nine calories. So, 15 grams of fat provide 135 calories. Alcohol interestingly falls between fats and carbohydrates at about seven calories per gram. Depending on our size, activity, and lifestyle, we need 1100 to 2500 calories per day to exist and keep our bodies functioning well (our resting energy expenditure requirement).

If we are gaining weight, we are either eating more calories than we need or utilizing fewer calories than we consume. Weight gain can also be caused by having a metabolic or hormonal issue that decreases our usual resting energy expenditure. Other reasons for weight gain occur when we have an underactive thyroid or an overactive adrenal gland, which can occur after significant weight loss, as the result of taking certain drugs, and when we are stressed or not sleeping.

On average, it takes 3,560 calories to gain a pound. Thus, eating just 100 extra calories per day, above what you need, for 35 days would result in gaining an extra pound of body weight. Examples of how this could happen are: if you change your eating pattern on a daily basis by adding a pat of butter, an extra slice of bread/mini-bagel, or by adding flavored syrup or cream to your latte. This tiny amount of extra daily calories can add up over a month. Knowing this is helpful if you are trying to lose weight. If you decrease your calories by 100-calories per day by cutting out your evening or afternoon snack, you will likely lose close to a pound in just over a month's time. Small daily changes either way result in large long-term changes.

Why Calories Are Not Just Calories & the Reasons Women Gain Weight

Calories are not always absorbed and used by the body in the same way over time. Many other factors can contribute to how the nutrition we receive is absorbed and used by our body. This is particularly true when we go through hormonal changes or stressful transitions in life. Some of these transitions also affect our activity and sleep. Women are affected by weight gain more so than men. We are affected by multiple hormonal changes as we go through puberty, pregnancies, and menopause, and we are more likely than men to have thyroid imbalances. These shifts can have a significant impact on our metabolism and our weight. For example, a typical concern I hear from my female patients is, "Oh my God! I'm gaining weight. I'm doing nothing wrong. I'm eating the same healthy things I ate before, even less, and yet I am gaining weight and feeling hungry."

What causes this kind of weight gain that frustrates so many women?

1. **Stress** is a primary cause. When women hold jobs that require a higher degree of responsibility and/or demand more time, they may not change what they eat, but experience more stress, are less active, and sleep less. Stress activates the adrenal glands to secrete hormones like cortisol and adrenaline. These hormones diminish the body's capacity to metabolize and use calories efficiently. We actually have a decrease in resting metabolic rate when we are stressed. Further, we tend to crave soothing comfort foods when we are in emotional angst. Learning stress reduction techniques to manage our stress or having a self-care practice is very important. Resting and breathing practices connect us to conscious awareness and the essence of who we are. Implementing stress reduction practices reboots our inner computer and expands our capacity to respond better.

2. **Inadequate sleep** increases appetite and cravings. If we don't get adequate sleep, a stomach hormone that increases hunger becomes elevated. Some of us eat when we should be sleeping, and these foods get metabolized in a way that is not optimal for our wellness. The resulting weight gain can be prevented or lost by making dietary changes, keeping a regular sleep-day cycle, prioritizing sleep, and aiming for at least seven hours of sleep a day. A beneficial habit that prevents the brain from worrying is to take the time to plan out the next day before going to sleep. Lastly, have 30 minutes of quiet and one hour away from computers or phones before going to bed.

3. **Hormones:**
   - *Estrogen*: Another cause of weight gain relates to changes in hormonal levels during menopause. As discussed above, menopause causes us to burn less calories per day with the same diet, and this frequently causes unwanted weight changes. The microbiome also changes as a result of estrogen deficiency, so we are more likely to get leaky gut because the altered bacteria do not make as much butyrate, which protects the gut lining. Fortunately, small changes in activity levels, calories consumed, and increased fiber in our diet can help counteract the effects of estrogen deficiency.
   - *Thyroid deficiencies* are common in women, particularly in midlife. If you experience weight gain, verify that your thyroid is working well. Ask your doctors to check your thyroid stimulating hormone (TSH) levels.
   - *Adrenal overdrive* can also result in weight gain. This may be caused by stress, depression, sleep deprivation, or tumors of the adrenal or pituitary glands. If managing stress and improving your sleep hygiene don't improve your weight management, ask your doctor to evaluate your adrenal hormones.

4. **Puberty** is a common and natural time for weight gain to occur. During this time, young women start menstruating and experience a normal increase in weight of about 18 percent (fat and bone mass) to create their adult weight. Estrogen, a hormone that comes from the egg-producing follicles of the ovaries, increases just around the time that menstrual cycles begin. Increased estrogen levels signal a young woman's body to begin physically changing, growing and developing more fat cells in the hips, breasts, and thighs in preparation for becoming fertile. Women's ancestral brains require a certain amount of body fat for the body to feel safe to get pregnant. A healthy diet and active lifestyle during this time create healthy weight gain in adult women.

For me, the excessive rather than the typically expected weight gain that I experienced as a teenager was caused by the "lethal triad": stress, sedentary lifestyle, and hormonal changes. I dealt with the high amounts of stress as a young immigrant by overeating the wrong foods, and my parents, in an effort to "protect" me, imposed a sedentary lifestyle upon me by keeping me close to home. The combination of overeating and lack of activity occurred at a time of hormonal changes when I was naturally developing more fat cells.

Through my education, I gained a better understanding of what led to my rapid weight gain, the resulting metabolic changes, and the subsequent negative psychological impact of becoming obese. This awareness allowed me to heal myself. I had been extremely self-critical about becoming obese. When I realized I was a victim of challenging circumstances and a lack of knowledge, that becoming obese was not my fault, I began to develop more compassion towards myself. This heightened awareness helped me guide my young daughters so they could have a healthy weight gain when they transitioned to womanhood. Many of the young women I have treated in my practice have also benefited from this knowledge.

Choose Good-For-You Carbohydrates

Carbohydrates, one of three major nutrients that fuel our body's cells, are often misunderstood, even vilified and vehemently avoided. The fact of the matter is that we need carbohydrates. Our bodies break down carbohydrates into glucose, or blood sugar, the main source of energy for our body's cells. There are two kinds of carbohydrates—simple and complex. Simple carbohydrates have been stripped of fiber and nutrients through processing or refining. Complex carbohydrates, however, are nutrient-dense and filled with fiber. We benefit from adding complex starchy vegetables in addition to non-starchy vegetables and fruits into our diet. Starchy whole food vegetables are great for the microbiome. We just need to limit them if we have insulin resistance, diabetes or want to lose weight.

The best way to appreciate what kind of carbohydrates are healthy is to understand the glycemic index (GI). The GI measures how fast the blood sugar goes up after we eat a carbohydrate. All carbohydrates, whether non-starchy (most vegetables and fruits) or starchy (carrots, peas, white and sweet potatoes, beets, yuca, plantains), increase blood sugar to some degree. This is expected and normal. However, some increase blood sugar more than others. Simple-refined carbohydrates (or processed carbohydrates) like bagels, pasta, chips, or boxed cereal have GIs greater than 50. Pure sugar has the highest glycemic index of 100.

Food with glycemic indexes greater than 50 cause a rapid rise and a higher peak in blood sugar levels. This occurs because these foods are highly processed. Refined grains, for example, have been ground into flour and are therefore "pre-digested" and more easily absorbed by the body. Since there is little to no fiber, sugar rushes into the bloodstream, and blood sugar spikes then drops quickly, which is why we often feel tired shortly after eating a processed carbohydrate. Non-starchy vegetables have a low glycemic index of less than 50. These vegetables have more fiber and fluid than starchy vegetables. The body digests and absorbs these complex, fiber-rich, and antioxidant-filled carbohydrates more slowly, so the entrance of sugar into the bloodstream is more gradual, resulting in a blood sugar rise that is not as high. Examples of these healthy veggies are leafy greens (collards and kale), asparagus, broccoli, brussels sprouts, cabbage, cauliflower, bok choy, peppers, zucchini, and celery, among others.

Eating whole foods is the healthiest way to get our carbohydrates. This is better for our bodies and better for our metabolism. We benefit our health and increase our energy when we stick to eating carbohydrates in the form of fruits, vegetables, and unprocessed whole grains.

Reverse Cravings, High Insulin & Diabetes

While we all need sugar, or glucose, to survive, we live in a day where many individuals struggle with abnormally high blood sugar levels. Diabetes, a disease in which blood sugar levels are too high, impacts millions of people. To fully understand these diseases, we need to understand the hormone insulin.

Insulin, a hormone made in the pancreas, is necessary for our survival. Insulin controls the amount of sugar moving throughout our blood and into our cells, where it is used for energy. Insulin is secreted in response to the carbohydrate content of our meals. The faster and higher blood sugar rises, the more insulin we need to process the meal and bring our blood sugar back to baseline.

Insulin also helps store glucose as glycogen in the liver for later use when we are fasting. The liver can hold enough glucose supplies to last about 12 hours. This short-term energy reservoir helps to keep our blood sugar (glucose) in a healthy range when we are not eating or engaged in serious exercise.

Glucagon is another hormone from the pancreas. It senses when our blood sugar levels are decreasing below normal and tells the liver to break down glycogen stores and release glucose so our blood glucose levels are normalized. This glucose is used by our mitochondria to create energy as we need it in all parts of the body, such as our muscles.

Years ago, when I used to run marathons, I learned the power of my liver's energy storage capacity when I would "hit the wall" at the 20th mile of the run because my liver had exhausted its glycogen stores. In those days, marathoners would drink water but not take nutrients. Now people routinely take in calories during these 26.2-mile runs.

There are two types of diabetes. Individuals—children and adults alike—who have type 1 diabetes lack insulin. When their blood sugars reach a high range, individuals with type 1 diabetes are unable to use glucose to create energy from food. This is extremely dangerous and can only be treated by providing the body with insulin. Individuals with type 1 diabetes require daily insulin injections or infusions in order to thrive. Unfortunately, not all people who need insulin have access to it. I am an advocate for insulin accessibility. I believe that insulin, an essential hormone, should be widely accessible and reasonably priced.

Individuals diagnosed with type 2 diabetes have insulin levels that are abnormally high. Despite producing a lot of insulin, the pancreas cannot produce enough insulin to keep blood sugars in the normal range. There is a resistance or a blockade to insulin's capacity to help the liver store glucose. The body determines that more insulin is needed and the pancreas secretes more insulin. However, the insulin-producing cells of the pancreas and their mitochondria are working overtime and eventually tire out. Toxicity from having high glucose levels too much of the time also burdens the pancreas and the rest of the body.

Healthy individuals, when not eating, don't have high insulin levels. Healthy individuals rely on stored energy from their liver and fat. If we have high insulin levels in the blood all day long, when such levels would normally be low from not eating, or after a night's fast, then we have a problem. This condition, called hyperinsulinemia, occurs when we have too much insulin in our blood stream. The liver, pancreas, and brain sense that nutrients are not being processed correctly, so the body keeps trying to put blood sugars and fatty acids from nutrients in storage, even if we have not eaten. This means we are not able to utilize the energy we have stored, because the body is actively trying to store even more. No matter how hard we try, we cannot lose weight.

Millions of people are diagnosed with conditions related to weight gain that cause higher blood sugar and insulin, such as metabolic syndrome, fatty liver, pre-diabetes, or type 2 diabetes. Yet most people do not know that weight gain is the origin of their condition or that this occurs as a result of the diet and lifestyle we have. This is particularly lethal, if we are sedentary and routinely have multiple meals or snacks containing refined or factory processed carbohydrates, refined or artificial sugars, and factory altered fats.

Over the years, I have met many individuals who struggle with serious effects caused by too much insulin. A high and continuous elevation of insulin in the blood can make our kidneys retain more salt and water, so we feel puffy, look swollen, and may have increased blood pressure. High insulin can also cause changes in the skin, so one can develop more skin tags around the neck and velvety dark areas behind the neck, armpits, elbows, knuckles, and knees. In addition, too much insulin negatively affects how our brain's nerve cells metabolize amyloid precursor protein; the more amyloid protein accumulating in our neurons, the more our risk for cognitive decline and Alzheimer's disease increases. I have served many women who have experienced damage to their ovaries and egg-producing follicles from too much insulin. Excess insulin, excess male hormones, or both are major causes of polycystic ovary syndrome (PCOS), a condition associated with irregular menstrual cycles and infertility.

So, what can we do to prevent and/or deal with the many numerous effects of these conditions: weight gain and obesity, high insulin, pre-diabetes, and diabetes? The first and simplest approach is to focus on our nutrition and choose the right foods for us. Secondly, we benefit from understanding the ancestral brain, and our tendencies to be drawn toward sweets and any available food to satisfy our cravings. The ancestral brain experiences a sensation of reward when we eat sweets due to the dopamine boost such foods provide. The release of dopamine is pleasurable and causes the brain to seek more rewards and increases cravings that we interpret as hunger. This causes us to respond by seeking more foods we don't need. Understanding the ancestral brain's agenda and its food cravings is important. If we are not aware, we will find ourselves struggling to say *no*, avoid, and eat less food than we actually need.

The medical community has realized that people regain weight after losing it because we have ancestral drives that *make* us regain weight. Most people are unaware of what is happening to them other than knowing they are hungry. There are medical treatments for obesity as well. Bariatric surgery helps address obesity, diabetes, and the risk of heart disease. There are also very effective medicines (incretins) that decrease appetite and improve metabolism and decrease weight. However, as a frequent prescriber of these medicines, I have observed that, a majority of the time, these medicines are not paid for by insurance and remain inaccessible. In addition, manufacturing companies have problems with production, sometimes running out of the drugs. Some individuals helped by the drug lose access to the beneficial effects due to insurance changes and loss of coverage.

Therefore, we need an alternative sustainable plan. We need to learn to rely more on ourselves, not outside sources. I want you to know that it's possible for each of us to respond effectively to our old ancestral brain cravings, body adaptations, and metabolic memories. It takes consciousness and effort to adjust our thinking and behavior to support our health and sustain a healthy weight. This approach can enable us to avoid drugs and surgery.

Our empowerment comes when we realize our ability to make choices about what and when we eat. We don't have to act upon cravings and hunger, particularly when we are trying to lose weight to prevent, manage or reverse diabetes, decrease the risk of heart disease, fatty liver, and cancer recurrence. Learning to not respond to cravings and hunger is hard to do at first, but this process becomes easier over time. When we experience hunger, we can remind ourselves that we will not die. Both hunger and cravings are transient sensations. We can utilize the energy deposits in our fat cells instead of eating every time we have a craving or feel hungry. This advice, however, does not apply to very lean individuals, or those with eating disorders which require a different approach for healing.

One of my patients lost 25 pounds over six months by applying these concepts. She learned to notice when she felt hunger cravings and then offer an agreeable nod. "OK, liver do your thing, use my fat for energy," became her new response instead of panicking and running for the food.

In summary, the key points to remember are that we need nutrients, oxygen, and water to make energy for our bodies to work. Nutrients from the foods we eat are broken into proteins, carbohydrates and fats. Insulin, a hormone crucial for our survival, helps our body function well by bringing broken down nutrients to the mitochondria in order to make energy. Too little or too much insulin causes significant problems in the body.

The type of foods we choose can heal or hurt us. What we eat and the frequency of our meals affect how much our blood sugar and insulin rise. The higher the blood sugar and insulin, and the higher the frequency of these rises, the more we exhaust our liver and mitochondria and store fat in the wrong places. This leads to inflammation and oxidative stress. If we choose inflammatory foods, we create more inflammation. Our cell's mitochondria make less energy and we age and get diseases faster.

What's amazing about metabolic havoc is that it can be prevented *and* reversed. We can make healthier food selections in our homes and our children's schools. We can decrease the amount of food we eat. We can reduce the frequency of our meals. By doing this, we can lower our insulin levels. Having normal insulin levels is one of the key components to aging slower and achieving our best health and vigor for our lifetime. I know this as a doctor, just as I know this from my own, human experience. I have followed these tips for decades now. I learned to talk back to my cravings and ignore them until they stopped bothering me. I have found that one meal a day is enough for me. Implementing these tips allowed me to achieve and sustain a healthy weight.

Contrary to popular opinion and what your ancestral brain wants you to believe, being a little hungry every day is actually good for you. Not acting on hunger for long periods of time, such as during intermittent fasting, awakens the innate healing capacity of one's body to lower excess insulin, normalizes how insulin works for us, and how our liver responds to insulin and our stored fat. This halts further unwanted weight gain and with time, prevents and reverses weight gain and diabetes.

Environmental Chemicals, Processed Oils & Artificial Sugars

Environmental chemicals can disrupt hormone actions and endocrine organs and promote weight gain. These chemicals can be found in plastics, beauty products, fuel, and even certain foods like soy. There is a valid concern that chemicals, like pesticides, are used to grow some of our food, such as mass-produced grains often used in processed foods. These chemicals directly damage the intestinal lining, possibly causing leaky gut syndrome. Leaky gut syndrome leads to body inflammation, autoimmunity, and cognitive decline.

Factory-produced foods often contain processed ingredients like fully or partially hydrogenated oils and high-fructose corn syrup (HFCS). These are food decoys with ingredients that are harmful to us. High-fructose corn syrup or *corn sugar* is an example of something that negatively affects our bodies and minds. HFCS, a processed sugar, differs from nature-made sugars like glucose, sucrose, or plain fructose from fruits. Unfortunately, this kind of sugar has become the predominant sweetener in most commercial and processed foods, such as salad dressings, syrup, and sodas. In general, sugars, especially those not natural to our body like HFCS, are "loved" by our ancestral brain, which experiences a reward sensation due to the dopamine boost they provide, and more cravings follow. These "sugars" also promote liver inflammation and prevent insulin from working well. To avoid sugars altogether, some of us choose artificial sweeteners, which have few to no calories. However, artificial sweeteners are also damaging. They disrupt the health and balance of helpful bacteria in the intestines. These chemicals, sugar-free or not, also activate the brain's reward systems, stimulating cravings that lead to weight gain. The calories you save by having the artificial-sugar-free sweetener might make you eat more calories than if you used regular sugar because of the excessive cravings they stimulate.

The food industry uses chemically-treated oils to create processed foods with a long shelf life. There's a saying, "the longer the shelf life, the shorter your life." Manufacturers know factory-made food needs to last through the chain of distribution—the transportation of food, the warehousing of food, the placement on shelves, and at long last, the purchase of the food by the consumer. Because manufacturers want food to last longer, they use refined or hydrogenated oils. None of these are good for us. These oils become rancid polyunsaturated fatty acids and trans fats over time. Rancid oils cause oxidative stress and inflammation that damages our cells, blood vessels, telomeres, and mitochondria. Trans fats increase our risk for heart attacks, strokes, and Type II Diabetes. However, we all benefit from foods that contain healthy fats from nature, like nuts, seeds, olives, and avocados. Unprocessed or freshly pressed oils, like olive, avocado or coconut oil, are healthier and safer.

A Few Words About Meat & Plants

The meat industry is the largest segment of the food industry in the industrialized world, with more than 25 billion pounds of meat being produced in the United States annually. Most people tend to eat meat from animals raised in crowded conditions with limited movement, which fattens them up faster. These animals are fed grains, such as corn, wheat, and barley, and treated with growth hormones and antibiotics. In humans, crowded conditions, limited activity, and a grain diet can make us inflamed and sick. Similarly, animals that experience these conditions likely have metabolic syndrome and inflammation that remain in their tissues. We, the consumers, might be eating and metabolizing these stressed and inflamed tissues. This is an avoidable inflammatory insult to our already compromised health.

I recommend that if you choose to eat meat, purchase meat that comes from animals that are grass-fed and free-roaming. The living and feeding conditions optimize the quality and type of nutrients we receive. Meat from grass-fed animals is less inflammatory for the body compared to meat or butters from animals fattened by grains. Grass-fed animals have less body fat and more of the healthy fatty acids our bodies need, such as the omega-3 polyunsaturated fatty acids and contain antioxidants such as glutathione and vitamins A and E, that are best for heart and body health. Grass-fed animals cause less metabolic stress to our bodies. This choice, though it is the more expensive one, is an investment in your health.

Another option attracting the attention of more people is to adopt a plant-strong diet. Substantial data demonstrates that populations with plant-based diets have a lower risk of cancer, heart disease, and Alzheimer's disease. This evidence is a strong incentive for us to decrease meat consumption. The average American eats 57 pounds of meat per year, three times more than people in other countries. *Estimating impact of food choices on life expectancy: A modeling study,* published in PLOS Med in February 2022, shares the findings of a meta-analysis using large data sets from the United States, China, and Europe. The study looked at life expectancy in relation to diet. They determined that life expectancy increases when people switch from the typical Western diet to a diet rich in fruits, vegetables, legumes, nuts, whole grains, and fish. Even if a person decides at the age of 60 to adopt a plant-strong diet, they can extend their lives by 8 to 9 years. Making the change at the age of 80 results in three additional years of life. It's never too late to improve your diet, but there are greater life expectancy gains with an earlier start.

Switching to a plant-strong diet can also ease the burden on our planet and lower greenhouse gasses (GHG). Cows are the number one agricultural source of greenhouse gas worldwide. Beef production contributes 25 percent of all food-based greenhouse gas emissions. Meat and dairy represent 14.5 percent of all man-made greenhouse gas emissions globally and 3 percent of all the US greenhouse gas emissions. A plant-based diet could cut these emissions by 63-70 percent. Greenhouse gasses contribute to environmental and physical health problems, such as respiratory diseases like asthma, chronic obstructive pulmonary disease (COPD), and other respiratory tract infections. Since a plant-based diet can cut greenhouse gas emissions significantly, it stands to reason that we'd see an improvement in our environment and health.

My Loving-Kindness Wish for You

May you have the wisdom to feed your body well
May you know what you need and when you need it
May you be increasingly discerning.

Meditation to Enhance Your Journaling

Please scan the QR Code with your Smartphone
or follow this link: https://youtu.be/JJvvKMSR7Os

Journaling for Transformation

Consider giving your pancreas and liver a break by eating less and having longer periods between meals. How frequently are you having meals and snacks? Have you developed a routine for this pattern of eating? I assure you: creating a new pattern of eating is possible if you put your mind to it.

1. Make a list of your top five foods. Are they all processed and sweet? You have an opportunity for improvement here! Choose whole foods and eat a more plant-based diet. Avoid machine-processed or refined foods whenever possible.
2. A whole food is just the food itself; nothing is added—no sugar, no salt, no preservatives, no additives. You can cook a meal and feel very good if you make half your plate filled with vegetables (not nutrient-deficient iceberg lettuce). Make a list of whole foods you are willing to add to your daily nutrition.
3. Did you know that sodas you buy, or mixers, are often sweetened with high fructose corn syrup (HFCS)? Even energy drinks contain HFCS. Your sweets should come from fruit. Select and eat fresh fruit rather than refined

or artificial sugars to keep your blood sugar levels in the normal range. Take inventory of your foods. What foods contain HFCS? Make a list of fresh fruits you can add to your daily food choices.

4. Ask yourself, do you REALLY need snacks between meals when you ate less than 2-4 hours ago? Especially if you are generally sedentary, sitting at your job all day rather than training for a marathon or triathlon. When you get the urge for a snack, ask yourself, "am I really hungry? Does my body need food now?" Open your journal and write.

5. Demonstrate and prove to yourself that you can survive if you skip indulging in one snack, then two snacks, then all snacks. After you do this, consider skipping a meal, I guarantee you will survive even if you are diabetic on insulin. In the latter case, you will actually need lower insulin doses—you just need the right amount, not too much. Take note in your journal of the challenges and benefits of skipping snacks and perhaps a meal.

6. Try not eating for 12 hours to allow your liver to give your body the nutrients it has stored. Do this for a few days, or a week, by not eating from 7:00 p.m. to 7:00 a.m. Take note in your journal of how you feel and what happens to your weight.

7. Take note of what and when your mind is craving particular foods, or focused on engaging in nonproductive activities. Ask yourself if you really need what your mind and thoughts are focused on eating or doing. Write about this.

8. Practice taking control and talking back to your mind. When you crave something, take 1-2 minutes before getting what you want. Ask yourself, do I need this now? And, what am I really feeling? Am I really hungry or just feeling angsty? Say *no* to the food cravings and activities that you don't need. Your ability to turn away from cravings and activities that don't serve you will become better the more you practice. Reflect in your journal on these questions and the transformation and empowerment you experience.

9. Consider taking a minimum of five minutes every day to focus on breathing, feeling your body, and finding gratitude. Take note of your breathing and somatic experiences. Keep an ongoing gratitude list. Notice how your life changes from these simple practices.

Chapter 5

Digestion & Gut Bacteria

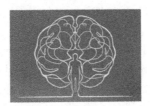

Our Miraculous Digestive System

What do you know about your body's digestive system? What organs are actually involved in eating and digestion? What happens after we eat food? How does food turn into nutrients that provide energy? How can we improve our digestion and elimination processes? Why is there so much focus on the health of our microbiome and gut health?

These questions and more allow us to explore and learn more about our amazing digestive system. It's time to fall in love with the miraculous processes of fueling our bodies and creating vibrant health.

Case Study: Ricky's Story

Ricky, a medical professional, first came to my office in her fifties with a recurrence of hyperthyroidism. She shared that when she was 30, she experienced jitteriness, weight loss, shaking hands, and diarrhea. She also suffered from joint pain. She was subsequently diagnosed with Graves' disease, an autoimmune condition that affects the thyroid gland. The body produces antibodies that bind to the gland and cause it to produce too much thyroid hormone. She was also diagnosed with celiac disease, another autoimmune disease where the body develops antibodies against gluten (wheat, barley, and rye), and as a result, the cells in the intestine become inflamed and stopped absorbing nutrients. At that time, she was treated with antithyroid medication and steroids, and adopted a gluten-free diet. She improved with her new diet. Her autoimmune flare-ups went into remission, her symptoms resolved, and her thyroid function normalized. When she visited my office, she was suffering again with severe joint pain due to the recurrence of Graves' disease. She had difficulty opening and closing her hands due to swelling. Her hands looked like bear paws; her knuckles were no longer visible. It became increasingly difficult to do her work which led her to retire earlier than she planned. Her arthritis doctor believed she had rheumatoid arthritis and was planning to treat her for this when her Graves' disease recurred.

Newly involved in her case, I began antithyroid medications and two anti-inflammatory supplements, curcumin, and omega-3 fatty acids. The thyroid levels improved; however, her diarrhea did not resolve. As a result of the persistence of diarrhea, despite a strict gluten-free program and now normal thyroid function, we decided to examine Ricky's stool to assess the bacteria in her gut. It was then that we discovered that Ricky had a few gut issues: small intestinal (bad) bacteria overgrowth (SIBO), low amounts and diversity of good bacteria, and leaky gut syndrome. Leaky gut syndrome, or gut permeability, allows bacteria to enter through the gut wall. This unwelcome entry activates an immune reaction to block the invaders from entering the rest of the body. This defensive reaction by the immune system causes inflammation throughout the body and can cause the onset of autoimmune conditions, such as Ricky had experienced.

Amazingly, three months after we began treating these conditions, the hand inflammation had resolved, and the joint pains disappeared. Her inflammation marker, C-reactive protein, went from 25 to 3, normal being 3 or less! We could see her knuckles again! The malaise she felt, from the chronic inflammation of her gut, resolved. She was now feeling more energetic and regained her weight. She could jog five miles a day again, and even her bone mass improved over the next two years. She now wished she had not retired! Her remarkable recovery from these inflammatory and immune-inducing conditions reinforced my opinion that, in addition to good food, normal function of the digestive system and having good gut bacteria are crucial determinants of health and wellbeing.

Essential Components of the Digestive System

As you can see in Figure 6, our digestive system is complex and requires the coordinated function of several parts, each playing a particular role that allows us to eat, digest, absorb nutrients, and eliminate indigestible remnants. Our digestive system contains smooth muscles which make synchronized contractions that transform the food we eat into nutrients that energize us and waste that is expelled from the anus. Let's review the individual parts of the digestive system to develop a better understanding of how they function and appreciate the magnificence of our bodies.

The Digestive System

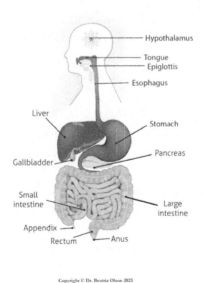

Figure 6: The Digestive System

Hypothalamus – A small area at the base of the brain that regulates hunger by sensing chemical signals sent from the stomach, our fat cells, and liver. These signals inform the brain about our relative nutrient supplies in these gut-related areas.

Tongue – The tongue is involved in digestion because it is involved in sensing, tasting, and chewing to break down nutrients and swallowing our food.

Epiglottis – Prevents food and liquids from entering the windpipe and getting into our lungs.

Esophagus – A muscular tube that transports food from the throat to the stomach.

Stomach – A muscular sac that churns and breaks down food further with enzymes and acids.

Liver – This amazing organ produces bile, which helps further break down nutrients as they enter the small intestine. Various toxins are metabolized and neutralized in the liver, and then excreted in the bile. The liver receives glucose and amino acids from the small intestine, and these are the nutrients used by the liver to store and make energy by the mitochondria. The liver makes essential proteins that help the body function well.

Gallbladder – Stores bile, the liquid produced by the liver, and passes bile into the small intestine to aid with the digestion of foods.

Pancreas – Creates key digestive enzymes, or juices, to support the breakdown of fats and proteins. The pancreas also makes hormones like insulin and glucagon, among others, which help our body utilize sugars to produce energy throughout the body.

Small Intestine – The small intestine further breaks down food coming from the stomach, absorbs most of the nutrients from these foods, and aids in pushing down fiber and waste into the large intestine. Trillions of bacteria live in the small intestine and help digest nutrients and communicate with the brain. The small intestine also makes hormone-like substances called incretins that communicate with the pancreas and other parts of the digestive system and brain.

Large Intestine – Absorbs water and salts from matter that has not been digested or absorbed in the small intestine and turns this matter into stools.

Appendix – The appendix was more necessary for our ancestors and perhaps is not an essential organ today. In the past, the appendix was known to help digest tough matter like tree bark.

Rectum – The storage site for solid waste material before it is excreted. It connects the large intestine to the anus. The rectum signals the brain when there is stool to be evacuated from the body. This is what gives you the urge to move your bowel.

Anus – The opening in the body that eliminates waste material from the digestive tract. The anus consists of pelvic floor muscles and sphincters.

The Calming Vagus Nerve & Digestion

The vagus nerve is the collection of main nerves that regulate the parasympathetic nervous system. The parasympathetic system controls involuntary body functions, such as our heart rate, immune system, and, as we will discuss here, our digestion. The vagus nerve connects our brain and gut. When the vagus nerve is functioning properly, the communication between the brain and the gut flows, but if the vagus nerve is damaged or working less actively, as when we are stressed, communication is impeded and digestive problems, like irritable bowel, occur.

Both physical and psychological stress impacts the functioning of the vagus nerve. Conditions like diabetes, obesity, stress, all addictions, and various forms of trauma reduce the operation of this important nerve, which then negatively impacts our digestion. For example, we might feel the sensation of butterflies in our stomach when we are nervous or stressed, individuals taking narcotics or who use pain medications after surgery might experience constipation, or the physical or hormone demands on the body during pregnancy may cause nausea, vomiting, or gastric reflux.

In addition to being responsible for how our gut functions, the vagus nerve communicates to your brain everything related to digestion and the health of the bacteria inside the gut. Similar to how the brain knows what is happening outside us through our senses, the brain uses the brain-gut connection to know about the status of our wellness through signals from the stomach, small intestine, and other parts of the digestive system. All communicated through the remarkable vagus nerve. In fact, our moods can be affected by our diet, which alters gut bacteria and the nature of our gut-brain interactions.

There are a variety of holistic options for improving digestion by improving the functioning of our vagus nerve, which can become sluggish as we age or from excess stress. Anything that is calming to our nervous system will improve the function of the digestive system. Examples of these are meditation, exercise, humming and singing, massage and music. I also recommend gentle, circular motion massage with the palm of your hand in a clockwise motion on your abdomen. You can also do a circular kneading motion using the knuckles starting from the lower right of the abdomen and gently moving up to the upper right, then across the upper abdomen to the upper left side and continuing down to the lower left side. This increases the motility of the colon and eases constipation.

Benefits of Sensual & Slow Eating

Let's imagine that we are sitting at a table in our favorite restaurant. Our favorite meal has arrived. When we first see and smell the meal, we begin to salivate. We take our first bite, and as we start to chew, our saliva, which contains the enzyme amylase, begins to break down the carbohydrates. The slower we chew, the more we fully utilize our taste buds, savor the taste and effectively signal our brain to prepare to digest and accept the delivery of the food. Also, the more we savor and chew each bite, the less we need to eat to feel satisfied and full. This is because our body has more time to send digestive enzymes and hormones to the right places in our digestive tract. These enzymes and hormones help us digest our food, slow down the amount the pace of our stomach's emptying, so we get fuller faster. This allows nutrients to be fully processed before entering the intestines.

In contrast, if we shovel the food in rapidly, the brain and gut do not get the signals fast enough, so digestive enzymes and hormones are not secreted in time to help digestion. We only sense we are full when the stomach's stretch receptors send a signal to the brain that the stomach is *very* full and the receptors have stretched beyond normal range. If you regularly eat fast and until the stomach feels stretched, you are probably eating much more than you need.

Chewing our food completely and eating more slowly are secrets to good digestion and maintaining healthy weight.

Functions of Stomach Acids, Juices, Mucus, & "Bugs"

We all need stomach acid to help us break down and digest the food we eat. The stomach also has specialized cells in the fundus, the top part of the stomach that connects to the esophagus. These cells make the hunger hormone *ghrelin*, which informs the brain when the stomach is empty. When we eat, food goes down the esophagus to the stomach. Cells in the stomach secrete hydrochloric acid used to break down proteins into amino acids. The hydrochloric acid lowers the pH of the food mixture, called chyme, before it enters the small intestine.

Please note that if we have little or no acid, as when taking an antacid, we can't digest food properly. We need acid to break down and absorb nutrients like iron or calcium. Without stomach acid, foods get to the small intestine less digested. This mal-digested food can induce the overgrowth of certain bacteria in the small intestine. This causes bloating, gas, and belly discomfort. This form of irritation to the bowels is called small intestinal bacterial overgrowth (SIBO). to avoid SIBO and help digestion, chew your food well, eat more slowly, add oregano to your cooking, and consider adding a little cider vinegar or lemon juice when eating proteins. Lastly, consider taking yogurt or probiotics when you take antibiotics.

When the chyme enters the small intestine at the duodenum, the gall bladder and the pancreas secrete bile and juicy digestive enzymes, respectively. This combination of juices further breaks down proteins and begins to break down fats into a form that can be absorbed through the small intestine. If we are missing pancreatic enzymes, we cannot absorb fats well, possibly resulting in loose or floating stools. If this is happening, chew food well, eat more slowly, consider decreasing the fat content of your diet, and try adding digestive and pancreatic enzymes with your larger meals to see if this helps.

Most digested nutrients are absorbed in different parts of the small intestine, magical places where good alchemy and occasional craziness happen. The small intestine has hormones called *incretins* (Glucagon-like or Glucagon Insulinotropic peptides, GLP-1, or GIP). Incretins help the pancreas secrete insulin to improve nutrient processing and metabolism. Incretins also slow down how fast the stomach empties, helping us feel a sense of fullness more quickly. Incretins don't work as well as they should for individuals who have diabetes and those that struggle with obesity. Doctors now use incretins as medical therapy to treat diabetes and obesity. These new incretin therapies—whose branded names are Ozempic, Wegovy, or Saxenda—will be discussed in chapter 6.

Mucus in the gut is made by beneficial bacteria that live in our gut. These bacteria are called the microbiome. Mucus has several important roles. It acts as a protective inner liner or coat for the cells that line the gut. Mucus helps the right nutrients enter the body, prevents toxins and bad bacteria in the gut from entering, and serves as a lubricant to ease the passage of waste out of the body. Mucus is necessary to trap viruses and bacteria so they can't infect our bodies; this helps prevent over-activation of the immune system.

The portal vein transfers glucose (from carbohydrates) and amino acids (from proteins) from the intestine to the liver. The liver takes this glucose and uses it to create energy in the body. The excess glucose is then stored in the liver as glycogen for use as energy when we are sleeping and fasting. The liver can convert fatty acids from fat and use these to make energy, just as it does with glucose. This happens when we are fasting for extended periods. The liver makes important proteins from amino acids taken from proteins in our diet. When we eat too much protein, amino acids can also be converted into fat and stored or made into glucose for energy.

Fats are transported differently since they are structurally bigger and not water soluble. They travel through the small intestine's cell walls into the lymphatic system. The lymphatic system includes fluids from all over the body and from the intestines that contain and transport fats and other fluid into blood vessels that eventually reach the liver.

Another important note: excess fats can damage our bodies. Regularly consuming high-fat foods such as processed or fried meals, meats, and dairy will increase the fatty acids, cholesterol, and triglycerides floating around; this results in an increased chance of the formation of cholesterol deposits in our blood vessels. To avoid these hydrolyzed- and saturated-fats and fat-associated damage, some cardiologists recommend that patients, especially those diagnosed with heart disease, eat a whole food plant-based diet. According to Caldwell Esselstyn, M.D., eliminating animal fats can reverse heart disease. I highly recommend Dr. Esselstyn's book, *Prevent and Reverse Heart Disease: The Revolutionary, Scientifically Proven, Nutrition-based Cure.* Another great book, and a New York Times bestseller, focused on a plant-based diet to prevent and reverse heart disease is *Forks Over Knives: The Plant-Based Way to Health,* edited by Gene Stone.

After nutrients are absorbed, the residue leaves the small intestine and enters the large intestine. This residue is composed of indigestible fibers, departing gut bacteria, toxicities metabolized by the liver for discard, and lots of fluids. The large intestine is less acidic and without oxygen. The bacteria in the large intestine create fermented short-chain fatty acids, like butyrate, that protect the integrity of the cells in the wall of our entire digestive system. Part of the large intestine is the colon. Colon bacteria love fiber. Fiber from vegetables is a "prebiotic" because it helps beneficial gut bacteria thrive and supports the digestive system integrity. We can use prebiotics and probiotics to create healthy and supportive bacteria in our gut. This is very helpful if we have to take antibiotics used to treat bacterial infections. Eating lots of plants, fermented vegetables, and avoiding excess sugars and red meat can serve to improve our gut health. Eating a healthy whole-food diet allows our large intestine to function well and transport the leftover residue and toxicities to leave our anus as excrement.

More on the Magnificent Microbiome

Trillions of microbiota live in our intestines. These microorganisms are primarily bacteria. We need these bacteria for our health and well-being. In fact, they are with us from birth and acquired through our cultural diets and social life. Our microbiome, or gut bacteria, protect us from disease, support the digestion of our food, produce vitamins, and help our bodies to absorb nutrients.

There are key signs that indicate we have a healthy or unhealthy gut. A healthy gut has a good balance of various groups and families of bacteria. When we have a healthy gut, we think clearly, have vitality, and respond to stress in positive ways. We have regular bowel movements. However, if our gut is less healthy, we are not absorbing nutrients as well. There is less healthy mucus lining our intestines.

As a result, we struggle with energy, have foggy thinking, and react to stress in less favorable ways; we crave sugar and less healthy foods and experience a variety of physical problems due to inflammation.

What contributes to gut inflammation? Gut inflammation happens when the gut immune system gets activated by various environmental factors. Our genetics can also predispose us to be more likely to react to or be allergic or sensitive to gluten or other triggering foods, potentially putting us at higher risk of celiac or Crohn's disease. A poor diet filled with processed foods and ingredients that aren't even food can also result in gut inflammation. The use of herbicides and pesticides, like glyphosates, in food production does not serve our health. These can cause leaks in the integrity of the gut wall and create inflammation. For example, when the cells in the intestinal wall lose their tight connecting junctions due to all these environmental factors, they become separated, then toxins or fragments of gut bacteria enter in between the cells and move through the intestinal wall. This is called leaky gut. The gut immune system tries to block these invaders by creating an immune inflammatory response which causes further generalized inflammation and oxidative stress on the body. The activation of the immune system can trigger autoimmune disease and bowel illness. Leaky gut symptoms include diarrhea, headaches, fatigue, malaise, fogginess, joint pain, rashes, and fatigue. When the permeability of the wall is impacted, as it was for my patient Ricky, we experience illness, joint pain, and even the onset of autoimmune diseases, like celiac disease, autoimmune thyroid disease, and arthritis.

Antibiotics also damage the healthy bacteria in the gut, so overgrowth of offending bacteria can inflame the gut, and it can take several months before the microbiome is restored.

Some researchers and doctors are concerned about particular kinds of food and their impact on the gut. Dr. Steven Gundry writes about the negative impact of lectins on some individuals. Lectins are found in the skin and seeds of tomatoes, eggplants, peppers, and beans. In his book

Grain Brain, Dr. David Perlmutter explores the gut- brain connection. He has identified wheat and other grains as toxic substances, even if you don't have celiac disease, that causes body and brain inflammation, which accelerates aging and contributes to diseases like Alzheimer's Disease. This because ultra-processed grains cause high insulin, inflammation and metabolic distress to the brain. In fact, Alzheimers disease is now considered Type 3 diabetes, and the reason why individuals with cognitive decline benefit from ketogenic diets, that decrease insulin excess exposure to the brain, or from medications, like incretins GLP-1 and GIP, that improve metabolism and insulin sensitivity at the brain. I identify deeply with this issue because, like Dr. Perlmutter's father, my mother suffered from Alzheimer's disease. Her only illness was intermittent gut inflammation or colitis, which she received medicine for until she went into remission, only for it to recur soon after. No one told her to change her diet. I did not know what I now know, and it's too late for her.

Another disease of the gut is celiac disease, which is caused by eating gluten in those who are genetically predisposed. Gluten is a substance present in grains, like wheat, barley, and rye. People with this disease have an immune reaction when they eat gluten. They experience symptoms like diarrhea, gas and bloating, constipation, abdominal pain, and weight loss. Some individuals that do not have celiac disease may be gluten sensitive, but not allergic, and may experience joint inflammation when they eat foods with gluten. General routine tests are not helpful, unless you have a full-blown allergy to wheat or celiac disease.

Other ailments that directly relate to the body-mind or gut-brain connection are depression and anxiety, which are epidemic in our modern world. Diet and digestion provide the brain with information that alters our mood and can exacerbate these conditions. My thinking about the power of gut bacteria was transformed after I read the well-researched and evidence-based book, *Psychobiotic Revolution* by Scott Anderson. Anderson establishes that food and gut bacteria contribute to our state of wellness. Probiotics help us when we are not feeling well; commonly available products, like the yogurt or kefir, can help our gut and brain health and support us to feel better.

What are some additional solutions to these various gut ailments? Good, healthy bacteria and good wall integrity can be maintained by avoiding foods that may cause problematic inflammation. Some individuals give up dairy, eggs, wheat, or corn and notice positive changes. Eating foods that support the growth of good bacteria and mucus can serve our gut health. Try cooking non-starchy and complex vegetables, such as artichokes, shallots and leeks, yams, or plantains. You can also supplement your diet with amino acids like glutamine and butyrate to support re-establishing the integrity of the intestinal wall. It's also helpful to give the body time to heal with longer pauses between meals.

Lastly, I want you to know about two main types of gut bacteria that are involved in determining how much of the food you eat is absorbed. Firmicutes are the bacteria that thrive with processed fast food, sugar, and fructose corn syrup-sweetened drinks in the American diet. They love these foods, and therefore help your brain make you crave processed, fat-filled, and sweet foods. Everything you give them is absorbed. A predominance of Firmicutes, or obesogenic bacteria, is associated with weight gain.

Bacteroidetes, on the other hand, are the bacteria that can see a calorie go by and say, "I don't need you right now, I'm fine." Bacteroidetes thrive with a vegetable-rich, plant-based whole food diet. They protect us from pathogens and supply nutrients to other microbiotas.

Information from studies conducted on animals and humans serve to convince all of us of the importance of the microbiome and diet on your health, digestion, and weight. In animal studies, stool samples from a fat mouse were put into a skinny mouse's intestine. The results? The skinny mouse gained weight and took on the characteristics of the fat mouse. Alternatively, the stool of a skinny mouse was put into a fat mouse. The fat mouse lost weight.

In humans, studies revealed that some patients who developed intractable diarrhea after antibiotics due to the overgrowth of a toxic bacteria called clostridium difficile (CDIF or CD) were immensely helped by receiving a fecal transplant from a healthy person. These studies demonstrate the power of having good bacteria to prevent disease and that of targeted probiotics to fix microbiome imbalances that cause disease. Most exciting is that the FDA approved, for the first time, a medical probiotic that can address CDIF without having a fecal transplant from someone you don't know!

I am often asked by my patients which prebiotics and probiotics to use. The following is a short list of pre and probiotics that address common health problems (I am not paid by any of these companies). Prebiotics, like Saccharomyces boulardii, help feed the good bacteria in our intestines, which is important to maintain bacterial diversity. Yogurt and kefir restore a group of bacteria called lactobacilli, among other bacteria, which help improve digestion, constipation, and mood. Some probiotics need to be refrigerated. Some probiotics, like Hyperbiotics, have a special casing that allows them to get deeper into the gut, where they work better and help with weight loss. A probiotic blend found in a product called VSL#3 has been shown to decrease insulin resistance and decrease weight. For my patients with fatty liver, I recommend they avoid processed and sugary foods. Avoid the white foods—white sugar, white flour, pasta, bread, crackers and cookies. Instead, I recommend a whole foods, lower carbohydrate and glycemic index diet. If you like, enjoy a cup of coffee in the morning, as coffee is a protective antioxidant for the liver. Two supplements that may help are milk thistle and a probiotic containing Lactobacillus fermentum ME-3. For women with recurrent urinary tract infections, I recommend eating less chicken (which may be colonized by e-coli) and taking probiotics with Lactobacillus rhamnosus GR-1 and lactobacillus reuteri RC-14, found in a few brands specific for women. Given that our gut's microbiome affects our moods, I suggest for those of us with stress/mood issues and gut distress a unique probiotic combination containing Bifidobacterium longum 1714™ and Bifidobacterium longum 35624 made by the Microbiome labs.

Lastly, I want you to know that when we eat meat, eggs, and dairy, all of which have the amino acids choline and L-carnitine, the bacteria in our intestines convert the choline and L-carnitine into trimethyl amine oxide (TMAO). The liver then removes the oxide (O) and converts TMAO into TMA. TMA goes into the blood and increases the risk of clotting related to heart attacks and strokes. This is particularly damaging for patients with or at high risk for heart disease. Yet another powerful reason to limit or stop our meat consumption—grass-fed or not, in our diet.

We will continue to grow our understanding of the miraculous nature and workings of our digestive system and magnificent microbiome. Who knows, in the future, probiotics may be our new medicine. I encourage you to continue to increase your awareness and improve how you care for your digestive system so you can enjoy an energetic and joyful life.

My Loving-Kindness Wish for You

May you truly appreciate your gut
May you tend well your gut's bacterial garden
May your gut bacteria be kind and protective of you

Meditation to Enhance Your Journaling

Please scan the QR Code with your Smartphone or follow this link: https://youtu.be/Dpw_v0z0P4k

Journaling for Transformation

1. Now that you have read this chapter, what changes will you make in your diet?

2. Have you been diagnosed with a digestive ailment, like irritable bowel syndrome? Have you considered how your diet or stress may be contributing to this?

3. What does your gut feel like after you eat? Do you have bloating and pain after meals?

4. Describe the pace of your eating? Are you eating too fast so that you are not digesting your food well?

5. What do you do or take to enhance your digestion? Could you be missing digestive enzymes?

6. Could you have a predominance of bad bacteria or SIBO (small intestine bacterial overgrowth)? Your gastroenterologist can do a breath test to evaluate this. Or you could take a special stool test for this.

7. What symptoms do you struggle with that might indicate gut problems? Are you feeling inflamed, experiencing fogginess, or a sense of malaise?

8. Have you ever wondered if you might have an autoimmune disease such as Hashimoto's or Graves' disease? Jot down any symptoms that disrupt your daily life. Are you noticing arthritis, stiffness, or joint pain? If you have these symptoms, you may have leaky gut syndrome or gut permeability. Sadly, many conventional doctors tend not to believe that this is a real condition, but functional and integrative medicine doctors like me do. As you learned with my patient, Ricky, there are ways to resolve it.

Chapter 6

Getting a Handle on Fat Cells & Weight

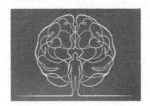

The Heavy Price of Obesity

In the United States, 70 percent of the adult population is overweight or obese. Obesity has health consequences that inhibit our physical and psychological wellness. Physically, excess weight and obesity cause diseases that age us faster and decrease our lifespan. These diseases include diabetes, high blood pressure, heart disease, cognitive decline, depression, and various types of cancer. Psychologically, excess weight and obesity contribute to suffering, frustration, and low self-esteem.

Most people who come to my practice are interested in losing weight and keeping it off. They have tried multiple diets that work transiently, but they tend to regain the weight they lost within two years, often weighing even more. As an integrative endocrinologist and a woman who dealt with a weight problem when I was younger, my professional mind understands my patients' struggles and my heart empathizes with them. My evaluation process includes figuring out who they are as people. I analyze lifestyle, habits, stresses and prior traumas, relationships, beliefs, pattern and quality of diet and sleep, activity level at work and home, exercise interests, and of course I check hormones like thyroid, insulin, and inflammation markers. A central part of this process is identifying the physical risks and psychological consequences that the weight problem poses. The higher the risks and severity of problems, the more we work to prevent, reverse or mitigate damage.

Nothing is more satisfying for me as a physician than seeing my patients succeed at overcoming weight problems and reverse diseases. These patients are successful because they are no longer willing to tolerate their weight problem and lack of health. They commit to uplevel their belief of what is possible for them to transform themselves for the better. They use new knowledge to overcome ancestral body-mind setpoints, and curiosity and compassion to overcome old habits and to manage the stress that in the past prevented their weight loss. They develop new self-care skills and beliefs that inspire lasting change.

Case Study: Jennifer's Story

Jennifer was 34 years old when we first met. Then she received a diagnosis of thyroid cancer requiring that her entire thyroid be removed, followed by thyroid hormone replacement. Though she had struggled with weight issues for years, her weight increased after her cancer diagnosis, despite taking higher doses of thyroid hormone— no doubt due to all the stress in her life. She had a demanding and stressful job as a social worker for a state department; she had lost two significant relationships within that 10-year period; her weight yo-yoed over the years.

During a recent office visit, Jennifer shared the following reflections on her health improvement and weight loss journey that occurred during the Covid pandemic:

> At the start of 2020 during the Covid-19 pandemic, I knew that I needed to make changes. I had a lot going on, and I didn't really take care

of myself. I took care of everybody else. I was about to turn 50 and suffered from inflammatory problems. My knees were killing me. I returned home from work every night with swollen legs from my knees to my ankles. I could barely walk. I went to many doctors who ordered blood work that ruled out different illnesses like lupus and rheumatoid arthritis. Yet my inflammatory marker c-reactive protein (CRP) was through the roof, and no one could tell me why.

It occurred to me that I had to take better care of myself. It was then during my office visit with you that you said to me, "You can change all this, with just the food you eat," I was ready to begin. I decided to eat smaller portions, eat fewer times a day, get a little more active. I even tried intermittent fasting. I started the day with the intent of just seeing how long I could go without eating. I didn't force a time. I didn't beat myself up. I kept healthy foods around so that when I ate, I chose vegetables and some fruit. I cut out carbs, pasta, breads, and cheese—things of that nature because I was ready to get my inflammation under control.

Within three to four months, remarkable changes occurred. I started feeling better. This was the biggest incentive to continue not putting all that garbage into my body.

Even though I didn't fast or eat perfectly every day and made mistakes along the way, I lost 120 pounds. I started at 350 and now weigh 230. That's a significant weight loss for me. I weigh less than I have most of my life, and I'm very happy about that.

I learned that it's not good to eat all that processed stuff. Now, when I do eat something that's not the healthiest, I don't even feel good. It's not worth it. I've developed a different attitude about food. I've learned that you have to eat to live and not live to eat.

When people ask me what's my secret, I tell them that there is none, and that I didn't have surgery. I just put less into my body. I stopped eating processed food from a box.

Dr. Beatriz, you had also talked to me about cortisol and stress. I truly think that my job was killing me. For the last two years, I have worked a much less stressful job. I have a set schedule. I know when I have to work and when I'm coming home. I'm not running around all hours of the night dealing with emergencies. I realized my personal lifestyle had to change. I had to learn how to decrease stress. Doing so and eating a better diet helped me. I feel so much healthier.

Jennifer illustrates how using whole food nutrition, smaller portions, longer intervals between meals, more movement, and lowering stress helped her use her body's fat cell storage to lose 120 pounds in two years. As we will discuss later, the task for Jennifer in the years and decades ahead will be to convince her ancestral mind-body unit that she is in fact not starving and that she is OK. This is everyone's task who loses weight and wants to sustain that loss.

How Do We Know We Have a Weight Problem?

While most people want to lose weight, many are unaware if they are truly overweight or obese. Many are often surprised to find out where they fall on the spectrum. Some are shocked and deeply saddened when they learn they are obese. While upsetting, this diagnosis can be very motivating for patients to make changes in lifestyle and weight. The World Health Organization and conventional medicine have two screening methods to define how overweight we are. The first is waist circumference and the second is body mass index (BMI). A waist circumference greater than 35 inches for women and 40 inches for men is consistent with obesity, and it carries a high risk of having heart disease or diabetes. This is because a large waist circumference reflects that a lot of the fat is inside the belly, where it should not be. This is called having an apple shape. Fat inside of the belly is inflammatory and damaging to our body, metabolism, and blood vessels. I invite you to calculate your risk using the Mayo Clinic BMI and waist circumference calculator:

https://www.mayoclinic.org/diseases-conditions/obesity/in-depth/bmi-calculator/itt-20084938

In contrast, people who have smaller waists, or are pear shaped, tend to store fat under the skin in the thighs, hips or arms. Fat in these areas does not cause inflammation, heart disease, or diabetes.

The BMI is the most commonly used screening method used by doctors and insurance companies to define your risk. It uses height in inches and weight in pounds to calculate body fat mass. A healthy BMI is between 18.9-24.9 for adults; an overweight BMI is between 25-29.9; an obese BMI is 30 and above.

Obesity is a disease condition of an extreme amount of body fat that puts individuals at risk for heart ailments and stroke, high blood pressure, digestive issues, arthritis, diabetes, and several cancers of the digestive system's organs, thyroid, kidney, and female organs. Most insurance companies use the BMI and the presence of other risk factors to define the risk of dying over time and decide if patients are sick enough by their excess fat to access weight loss medicines and treatments. The BMI, however, is not a perfect screening tool for fat mass because people who have a high muscle mass may measure as overweight or obese, and people who have very little muscle and large fat mass may be considered normal.

In addition to these two categories, *overweight* and *obese*, I have created a third category called *lack of wellness* in the normal weight domain. Many of my women patients desire to lose weight, even if they are technically not medically overweight. They don't feel well in their body. This is particularly true in women aged 40-65 during the pre-and post-menopause period. I aim to address this concern and reduce my patients' suffering. Weight gain, a shift in fat distribution, and a change in how our clothes fit as we get older, causes an enormous amount of psychological distress that, in my view, is equally important to address and mitigate.

While we addressed the management of this type of weight gain in Chapter 4, to more deeply understand our struggles with excess weight, we need to answer the following questions:

- Are you a normal weight, overweight or obese?
- Are your fasting sugars less than 100 mg/dl, insulin less than 5 mIU/L, and CRP less than 3 mg/L? If so, this is very good, if not you may try to improve them.
- Are your hormones in a healthy range for your age?
- Do you already have a weight-related disease like heart disease, high blood pressure, or diabetes? If you do, what are you doing beyond taking pills to mitigate or reverse this health condition?

Why Do We Gain Weight?

There are various reasons that we gain weight. Many of them are ancestrally set by our survival-driven physiology and are technically not our fault. Once these reasons are understood, they can be managed. Others are caused by an imbalance between the nutritional energy intake through diet and how much energy our body is using to run the functions of the body (the basal or resting metabolic rate). In general, weight gain happens when we consume more calories than we need or use.

However, there are times when we gain weight even when we are not overeating or changing our diet. In these situations, something has happened that has led to a decrease in our metabolic rate. Sometimes we have a combination of both overconsumption and decrease in metabolic rate, and this leads to rapid weight gain. In general, many of us are eating WAY too much and very few of us are aware of when our metabolism slows down or what causes it to slow down. The common things that slow down our metabolism are hormone deficiencies like estrogen, testosterone, and growth hormone; adrenal hormone excess of cortisol from stress, depression, sleep apnea or sleep deprivation; and endocrine conditions of adrenal or pituitary non-cancerous tumors, and rare pancreas insulin producing tumors. In addition, weight loss by itself slows down our energy expenditure too! Lastly, some medicines can slow down our metabolism. For example, antidepressants or antipsychotics for mood and psychiatric conditions, or beta-blockers for cardiovascular issues. Medicines like antihistamines and antipsychotics can increase hunger. Because some medications affect our weight, we can discuss the possibility of switching to more weight neutral medicines with our doctors.

While there are many reasons for weight gain, I believe the most prevalent cause of the excess weight problem is overconsumption. We all need to register that weight gain and obesity are not indicative of moral failure. The fact is that weight gain is not all our fault. We have unknowingly become victims of a biologic paradox. Over millennia, we developed fat cells to coat our bodies from the cold, ensure fertility, and help us survive famines by using our stored fat as energy. In contrast, when food was plentiful, our liver and metabolism were designed to shift into using foods found in nature as energy and storing the excess nutrition into our fat cells in preparation for the next famine. Nowadays we don't have famines, we just have food abundance. Yet our ancestral biology's need to ensure survival causes us to over-consume food. Unfortunately, we have not evolved to lose our appetite or stop consuming when we have excess fat.

Lose Weight & Keep it Off: Challenges & Solutions

Let's examine the biological and emotional reasons that make it difficult to lose and keep off excess weight.

Biology

Our ancestral brain is geared to hold on to weight to survive famines. We have not had any evolutionary adaptations to lose weight when we want to. The rates of obesity have dramatically increased over the last few generations, and it takes thousands of years for our metabolic biology to change as a result of environmental selective pressure. Worldwide, the rates of obesity have tripled over the last few generations. In America 1 in 4 adults are obese and, in many places, food is abundant. Even though many people desire to lose weight, the ancestral brain goes into a major state of alert when we lose weight. Evolutionarily, the brain is programmed to maintain the highest weight we have ever been, the brain's "defended weight," as a defense against famine.

The alarm system triggers more cravings to prevent further weight loss. Cravings are more intense than actual hunger. The food around us looks and smells more appealing than ever. We want it viscerally. The increased food cravings, and increased sense of hunger reflect our ancestral fear of not having prepared enough storage for a famine. This happens regardless of how much fat our body has. This is why we often cave into the cravings. We go back to eating the processed foods that caused the excess weight gain in the first place in order to satisfy the brain's ancestral anxiety about starving; this causes us to regain the excess weight we initially lost and, often, we gain a bit more.

Another factor that contributes to mitigating further weight loss relates to our resting metabolism, which slows down when we eat less and lose weight. In fact, when we participate in any diet program, we tend to lose 5-8 percent of our weight and then our weight plateaus. When we don't see the scale dropping, we feel frustrated, and this diminishes our efforts at weight loss.

We must develop consciousness and discipline to overcome the cravings and talk back to the brain when we are trying to lose weight. We must develop the skill of telling our brain we will survive without eating the treat we crave. When we do this, we are choosing to let our liver use its ancestral survival talent of getting all the energy we need from our fat cells. Many of my patients, like Jennifer, are amazed as to how they can continue to lose weight beyond expectations, once they choose the right foods and learn to mindfully override ancestral lack and survival-driven mechanisms. They reactivate their ancestral liver biology to use stored fat to give them energy while they lose unwanted weight.

Another way that our "defended" weight is guarded by each of our ancestral survival systems may have to do with the lifespan of the fat cell population present in the body. Consider that we don't lose fat cells when we lose weight. Rather, we shrink their volume. As mentioned, the mind-body units interpret the fat cell volume decrease as if it has entered a famine. I surmise that an additional part of our tendency to regain weight has to do with the cycles of replacement of our fat cells. Every cell in our body is replaced at different rates. For example, the cells that line our gut are replaced by new ones every few days. In contrast, fat cell turnover occurs very slowly. Only 8 percent of our fat cells are replaced every year, so it takes about 15 years to replace our entire fat cell number. Theoretically, if we were to lose weight slowly and keep a lower weight for 15 years, then perhaps, the ancestral mind-body unit might register that we are not in famine or survival mode.

Personally, I have maintained my healthy lower weight for two of these 15-year cycles. Through patience, long-term dedication, I have created a new setpoint. My body is comfortable with my past weight loss and my current weight. Through knowledge and conscious awareness of how my body and brain operate, especially awareness of how our ancestral survival system guards a "defended" weight, I have overcome my personal struggles with obesity and helped many of my patients do the same.

As you can see, there are biological and ancestral reasons why sustaining weight loss challenges us. Most people do not have access to this kind of knowledge about the biology of weight gain, so they cannot help themselves. When we lack understanding of what has to be done and how long this process will take, we cannot envision the patience and consciousness required to stay on course to lose and not regain weight. In general, only 10 percent of people that lose weight do so sustainably.

Emotions And Trauma

Separate from the realities of our ancestral brain biology and its tendency to hold on to our weight, I have frequently observed that our stress can sabotage our effort of weight loss and wellness goals. We often soothe these angsty states by eating, regardless of whether our bodies need more calories. I find that the stories younger parts of ourselves (inner family system) tell us based on prior traumatic experiences (see chapter 2) and the habits that have been developed to protect us from consequences of past stress, trauma and criticism (chapter 3) often block our ability to lose weight or sustain a healthy weight. As we discussed in the first part of this book it's important to take a mindful pause to be present and hear what the emotions are telling us about their inner suffering. Just as we can consciously talk back to our brain and do what we need to do to be healthy now, we can reassure inner younger parts of ourselves that fear the worst. We need to compassionately embrace and support inner anxious younger parts of ourselves that are either afraid that if we lose weight we will suffer, or that if we try to lose weight we will fail because we are fundamentally bad.

Outer trauma if we have been physically or sexually assaulted or the negative messaging that emotionally hurt us becomes internalized as shame. Shame leads to a sense of inadequacy and isolation. These feelings disempower us and result in chronic damage in all domains of life. To overcome these deep hurts requires higher levels of nurturing. Therapists and trauma experts can help process these traumas, which is essential for sustained weight loss.

Stress

Another factor related to emotional healing that affects our weight is how well we learn to manage stress. Stress, a feeling of emotional or physical tension, happens to us all. Stress can lead to a variety of difficult emotions, even physical tension and pain. Stress interferes with digestion and gut motility, metabolism of nutrients, and energy expenditure. Stress is inflammatory to our bodies.

Since stress is part of our life, and some stress beneficial, we don't always realize when our stress levels increase. We may just sense that we're not feeling quite right. Perhaps we're tired or a little bit irritable. These sensations activate the ancestral stress-management system and the fight-flight-freeze response. The ancestral-response system's job is to keep us safe and out of pain. When adrenal hormones increase, so does the signal to do something to escape the pain. A rewarding, rich sensory experience, like eating sweet or salty, processed carbohydrate-rich foods, can distract us from the pain and temporarily relieve the discomfort.

We can all learn about and implement healthy and compassionate ways to respond to stress, emotions, and angst. First, we can learn how to name and feel the variety of emotions that arise in us rather than escaping them through unhealthy means. We can learn to sit with the situation we are facing. We can take the time to acknowledge our feelings, interpret and make meaning of what is happening, rather than leaving our pain uninterpreted and meaningless. This does not need to take hours. Sometimes, a two-minute pause to reflect on a situation gives us the time we need to reframe our perspective and respond wisely.

Other ways to manage stress include going for a short walk, listening to music, moving, or dancing, engaging in art activities (even something as simple as doodling), calling a friend, writing in a journal, or listening to a self-help talk or guided meditation. These kinds of creative and growth-producing activities calm our nervous system and empower us to more effectively deal with the stress in our lives. All of these are calorie neutral and can counteract old patterns of eating, drinking, and numbing or ignoring difficult emotions. When we choose to manage stress in proactive ways instead of the old ways, a more empowered part of ourselves is regulating our caloric intake rather than our ancestral brain.

We can all develop self-awareness and grow. We can invite the most empowered and developed part of ourselves to take charge of our lives, rather than our fleeting thoughts and emotions. We can access the parasympathetic, or calming, nervous system by connecting to our breath to decrease the effect of stress on the body and soothe our emotions.

My short, guided meditations

(https://youtube.com/playlist?list=PLB2yiywncwdWlKNwreDZ4NO RLcsjhqWFb), or the meditations of others suggested in the Resources section of this book, can help ground us, and align our mind and body to our spirit's innate wisdom. The regular practice of these techniques can help us to identify and manage our many emotions so that they have less power over us and our choices.

Why Diseases Happen When We are Overweight or Obese

When we gain weight, we initially store the excess nutrients in white fat cells under our skin. The more we eat the wrong types of food, the more that we overwhelm the capacity of our liver and pancreas to process all these extra calories. The body makes more fat cells in order to store extra calories as fat. This fat gets stored inside of the abdomen between our organs, between muscles and our liver. An abundance of abdominal or visceral fat, as well as overstuffed fat cells, causes inflammation and metabolic havoc. Too much fat in the liver is called fatty liver. Similar to alcohol excess, too much fat in the liver can damage the liver and even cause cirrhosis and liver failure. Sadly, fatty liver afflicts an increasing number of younger people who are overweight or obese. The high levels of the storage hormone insulin and the inflammation caused by all these disenfranchised fat-filled cells causes incredible oxidative stress for the body.

The triad of high insulin, inflammation, and oxidative stress taxes our metabolic processing systems, damages our cell's integrity and diminishes the mitochondria's capacity to make energy. Damaged and old cells send signals of inflammation throughout the body. As a result, we feel tired. The inner lining of our blood vessels become unstable and fat and cholesterol deposit in these spaces, increasing the risk of heart attacks and strokes. The blood vessels become stiff and affect the kidney, resulting in high blood pressure. Our joints ache and flexibility and movement decline. All this ongoing inflammation shortens telomeres and interferes with DNA replication and cell division, increasing the risk of cancer.

Besides inflammation, insulin excess, and oxidative stress, high sugar in uncontrolled diabetes directly damages the pancreas. This metabolic stress causes damage to nerve cells in our brain and increases the risk of cognitive dysfunction over time. Too much insulin is also a common cause of polycystic ovary syndrome and infertility in women. The excess insulin interferes with the function of the ovaries and their egg-producing follicles, causing irregular periods, infertility, and the production of excess male hormones that cause acne and excess hair growth in unwanted areas for women.

Just as weight gain and obesity increase diseases, weight loss can decrease the risk for these diseases. These diseases can be prevented or reversed by eating whole, unprocessed foods; moving and sleeping more; and allowing our bodies, especially the liver, to naturally shift metabolism between periods of eating and periods of fasting.

Recently, I received an email from a friend reporting that he had made the dietary and lifestyle changes that my husband, Eric, and I had recommended after he shared with us that arthritis was seriously interfering with his career as a musician. He was having trouble playing the piano and guitar due to the pain and swelling in his fingers and hands. The prospect of this progressive and looming long-term disability had distressed him greatly. Our recommendations inspired him to eat more plants and whole foods and ditch the dairy creamer he added to his morning coffee. As a result of making these changes, he lost 15 pounds. The inflammation in his hand was reduced by 90 percent so he could resume playing his beloved instruments without pain. We were so happy for him to experience the healing properties of good nutrition.

How Much Weight Loss is Necessary to Improve Our Health?

You may be wondering how much weight loss is needed to make a difference in your health. Based on all the research data, for overweight individuals who wish to reverse disease, 5-7 percent weight loss improves overall quality of life by reducing blood sugar levels, depression, sleep apnea, and urinary incontinence. A 10 percent weight loss is required to measurably decrease heart disease risk. Greater weight loss of 15-20 percent may be needed to reverse diabetes in obesity. I'm happy to report that my patients who exercised discipline and patience achieved these higher percentages. They remained aware of the ancestral brain's cravings and adaptations and learned to not cave in to these cravings.

Despite our best efforts, some of us are unable to access, organize, initiate, maintain, or succeed at self-directed lifestyle or dietary changes that are designed to decrease the harmful effects of obesity-related diseases. For these individuals, weight loss of 25-35 percent is also achievable with the aforementioned pharmacologic incretin therapies and surgical bariatric procedures. There are two effective bariatric procedures: (1) gastric bypass is the best procedure to reverse diabetes, (2) and gastric sleeve, less invasive than gastric bypass, also reverses diabetes and can stimulate 25-35 percent weight loss. Most of this weight loss is observed in the first year after the procedure. As with all surgeries, there are risks. These procedures, particularly gastric bypass, can increase the potential for vitamin and nutrient deficiencies which can cause life-threatening conditions. Careful monitoring is required to avoid bone mass loss and nerve function complications. Replacement of vitamins and strength training can help counteract these effects. In addition, some patients who are emotional or binge eaters can regain their weight, despite the surgery. I have observed this over the decades I have cared for patients. I strongly recommend having therapy to address these eating disorders before considering bariatric surgery.

For many, weight loss medicines and surgeries are not an option. I know many people who do not desire to have bariatric surgery, even when it is recommended to them. I also treat many people with the new pharmacologic incretin therapies. However, sometimes these medicines become unavailable, or insurance coverage changes and the medications are no longer covered for the patient. This is why I feel strongly that, beyond what conventional medicine can offer us, we need to be skilled at overcoming our biological and emotional drives that prevent weight loss.

It is also important for people to be aware of the strategies used by the 10 percent of individuals who successfully keep their weight off after significant weight loss and without counting on the medical system to help them. Their strategies include the following:

1. Exercise most days, such as by walking 3-4 miles
2. Keep a fairly regular meal pattern, even on weekends and holidays
3. Monitor weight.
4. Eat and cook at home
5. Take time to create a meal plan
6. Set realistic, achievable goals
7. Keep healthy foods at home
8. Reduce consumption of carbohydrates
9. Increase consumption of protein
10. Chew more slowly and savor the food

When we combine these strategies, we will experience numerous benefits. We will feel better and enjoy the food we eat. We will avoid feeling deprived, sustain weight loss and prevent or reverse diseases.

My Story

As a freshman in an all-girls school, I wanted to develop skills to perform on the floor and balance beam, so I tried out for the gymnastics team. At one of the practices, the coach asked team members to reflect on our strengths. I recognized and shared that I was a flexible and muscular dancer. "You're not muscular; your legs are fat," the coach responded in front of all the girls, and laughed, causing everyone else to laugh. The humiliation felt like a heavy weight crushing my stomach, my throat, and my chest. I looked down at my thighs. They looked like thick tree trunks. At that moment, I lost my desire to be on the team. I started feeling critical of my legs and began to cover them. I became increasingly unstable on the balance beam. These few words heard at a vulnerable age altered my confidence, carriage, and body image for years.

Words carry great power, and critical words can impact us throughout our entire lives. In addition, the media's obsession with thinness and the anti-obesity cultural messages creates fixed mindsets about individuals who struggle with excess weight and obesity. Many of us, particularly women, are the recipients of direct or indirect weight or obesity bias. The pain of this bias can cause us to react in disempowering and life-limiting ways. We may turn inwards and become critical of ourselves—jailed by perfectionism. We can become invisible, hide our talents and gifts, losing the capacity to be fully seen by others. We can struggle with anger and frustration, often giving up or sabotaging our efforts to be healthier. We can stop making efforts to live a healthier life, which unconsciously reinforces our inner sense of failure and shame. We may even deliberately, as an act of rebellion against the media, work to maintain our obese state. All of these responses to fat shaming are physically harmful, and increase our risk of weight-related diseases and limit our possibilities of achieving self-acceptance and a more joyful life.

There are functional ways to get out of these negative spaces. I have been able to do this and helped others do the same. The healing requires greater connection to our bodies and awareness of our bodies' innate healing capacity. We need to consciously embrace the truth that we are inherently worthy—regardless of anyone's opinion or cultural bias. We must befriend ourselves and tend to our needs, behaviors, and emotions with compassion and loving acceptance. We need to treat ourselves as we would treat a child we love who is facing this body-mind problem. I believe that if we better understand our bodies and the process of weight gain, we will be more compassionate with ourselves and others.

For me, practicing compassion towards myself healed the criticism I had internalized from those early days of gymnastics practice. Instead of disliking and hiding my legs, I am now thankful for the mobility and independence they provide. The greatest gift we can give ourselves is to allow ourselves to feel grateful for our bodies, regardless of what weight we have. This type of mindset helps us make health decisions based on our authentic desire to be physically healthy rather than on outside opinions of how we should look and be.

Conventional Medicine: Obesity & Solutions

Conventional medicine recognizes obesity as a disease that causes illness and decreased life expectancy. Obesity is also incredibly expensive to manage. Most doctors now understand the biology of ancestrally driven weight gain and hunger. We understand that our patient's obesity plight and tendency to regain weight after weight loss is not due to moral failure: it is due to an ancestral biologic drive to survive gone awry in a world of food abundance and no famines. Physicians now use new and effective drugs that target the metabolic derangements that keep us eating when we are obese. These medications mimic incretin hormones (see chapters 4 and 5) in our digestive system. They help decrease appetite by improving the digestive and metabolic dysregulations directly in obese and overweight patients with cardiovascular risks or diseases. I believe they can help overweight patients, like my patient Jennifer, who do not have obesity or diabetes to sustain weight loss.

Specifically, the new class of weight loss medications is called the incretins. Their genetic and brand names are liraglutide (Saxenda), semaglutide (Ozempic and Wegovy) and tirzepatide (Mounjaro). Each one, in order, is more powerful than the other in improving blood sugar and producing weight loss. For example, tirzepatide, at high doses, can induce a 20 percent weight loss. These drugs are powerful stimulators of insulin release; they slow down the way that the stomach empties, and as a result we get fuller faster. This reduces cravings and the desire to eat. The drugs also stimulate hormones involved in fat metabolism, promoting weight loss.

The negative and positive side effects of these drugs are associated with digestive issues like nausea, vomiting, gallstones, and in some rare cases, pancreatic inflammation. These medicines cannot be used in patients who have had or are at risk of medullary thyroid cancer.

They, however, appear to be safe for patients with autoimmune problems as the drugs do not appear to cause immune activation. The individuals taking these drugs who experience weight loss benefit from a decrease of inflammation and the many conditions associated with inflammation.

While I love these drugs, I have observed the medication will not work as well when individuals continue to habitually eat too much, especially if the foods are processed and artificial. In addition, the drugs are not always available, so it is crucial to change lifestyle habits and learn to eat healthy foods in smaller amounts. This awareness goes a long way to preventing the weight regain expected after you stop the medicine.

Bariatric surgery is another option to treat high levels of obesity. Two different surgical procedures adjust the digestive system so the patient can effectively lose weight. They are gastric bypass and sleeve gastrectomy. These surgeries assist patients with obesity to rapidly counteract risks and reverse diabetes. These procedures are very helpful and can cause up to 30 percent weight loss in one year but also have their own potential complications and potential for weight regain if emotional eating is not addressed. In the future, we may be able to offer increasingly powerful medicines and no longer need to do bariatric procedures. Currently, despite the documented need for these treatments, many insurance plans do not cover weight loss medications or surgery and these procedures or medicines are inaccessible in many communities.

The reason why I don't think these treatments are best is that we are not empowered to sustain our weight when they are not available. This is why I provide education on how to manage our ancestral brain and provide nutritional options for each of us to find our way to wellness.

Diets, Diets & More Diets: What I Recommend

The real definition of diet is our habitual eating and drinking pattern, our daily consumption. However, for many people a diet is associated with restriction, what we can and can't eat and drink to lose weight. These kinds of weight-loss diets work for a while because they transiently create dietary change, mindful eating, and lower calorie consumption. The dieter begins and holds themselves accountable to the diet but may not have realistic expectations around weight loss or understands that for dietary changes to work they must become habitual and part of their long-term lifestyle. It is realistic to expect weight loss with any diet of about 5-10 percent. Why not more? Remember that ancestral survival adaptations will hinder additional weight loss. Further, often when we enter these diets, we are not simultaneously addressing emotional aspects of our eating habits. When this happens, the normal response is to feel discouraged and effort-fatigued. We lose patience and may abuse ourselves with negative and demoralizing thoughts because we cannot follow through. Then we stop trying and give up. This is not helpful and keeps us in a state of non-possibility. It takes a lot of time, curiosity, consistency, self-compassion, and many small steps to get to be healthier when we are dealing with excess weight. The new knowledge and skills you have acquired through this chapter will help you overcome expected biological and emotional setbacks.

What if we were to consider adopting a plan of eating that nourishes our body and becomes a healthy way of life, rather than focusing on restriction? Let's explore the various options that exist and choose a more intuitive way of eating to fuel ourselves, honor our health, and that we can embrace as our lifestyle. Not all people need to lose weight or to focus so intently on weight loss. On the other hand, some people may appear normal weight but have low muscle and high fat mass and are metabolically unwell. Perhaps we could all focus more on caring for ourselves and giving our bodies the healthy foods they need to be well.

There are various eating plans, referred to as diets, available to us. I have seen my patients achieve successful weight-loss with a number of programs during the time that they participate with them. There are benefits to several diet programs. However, I feel that programs that address emotional aspects of our eating and emphasize eating whole foods and avoiding processed foods are more successful at preventing weight regain.

The **Mediterranean diet** has been studied the most and consists of whole foods, mostly plants, fish, nuts, and olive oil (a monounsaturated fat). The Mediterranean diet is generally low in saturated or commercially hydrogenated fats, which are inflammatory and cause cholesterol deposits in the blood vessels of the heart and arteries. It is a good choice, particularly for people at risk of heart disease. **Low-fat, plant-based diets** can be very effective at reversing heart disease, but a low-fat diet (less than 10 percent fat) is difficult to sustain long-term and decreases metabolism the most with weight loss. **Plant-based diets,** with adequate amounts of healthy fats, are associated with lower risks of cancer and heart disease. **Paleo-based diets** involve avoiding grains, dairy, and beans, including soy; this can be helpful to individuals dealing with autoimmune, inflammatory, or cognitive issues, where grain and dairy may contribute to the immune or inflammation problem. In general, a plant-generous paleo program helps most people be well.

Ketogenic diets are high in fat and limited to less than 30-35 grams of carbohydrates per day. These diets help individuals maintain a higher metabolism and resolve the problem of excess insulin so that the liver can use fat from the diet and fat cells as its energy source. The brain loves ketones as a nutrient source, so ketogenic diets are helpful to individuals with seizure disorders, cognitive decline and Alzheimer's, or those dealing with cancer who want to minimize excess insulin effects on tumor growth. Ketogenic diets are hard to sustain however. I find that my patients with cognitive decline are very resistant to dietary changes. Maintaining this type of diet requires long-term commitment and careful planning. Various keto-green books can be found online and in the resource section of this book that can support individuals with meal planning. If you choose this diet, I recommend using lots of olive or avocado oil, fish, and chicken, instead of dairy fat and red meat, as well as non-starchy vegetables as the carbohydrate source.

Recommendations for Patients with High Insulin, Prediabetes & Diabetes

Based on years of experience supporting high-risk, overweight, and obese patients to lose weight in order to decrease their disease risk, I tend to recommend a whole-food variant of a Mediterranean Diet, using vegetables as the carbohydrate energy source of this program. I also include increasing degrees of interval fasting periods, the higher the fat mass and the higher the insulin. This is particularly important for people who have been diagnosed with the following:

- Metabolic syndrome
- Fatty liver
- Prediabetes or adult-onset type 2 diabetes
- PCOS
- Cognitive decline
- Cancer

I advise these patients to cut out all refined sugar and processed carbohydrate foods. Period. These dietary changes can be life-saving and disease-reversing. Recent data suggests that having the largest meal earlier in the day leads to less caloric consumption during the day and lesser cravings, so I invite individuals to try this. Personally, that does not work for me or my lifestyle. I encourage a lower carbohydrate diet using veggies with a low glycemic index which aids in reducing fat-related inflammation and cancer-promoting effects caused by having excess insulin. Lower insulin and glucose levels let the liver, during fasting periods, remove fat from the wrong places and use that fat to produce energy. Also, when you consistently avoid processed carbohydrates and sweets, the microbiome changes, and cravings and hunger sensations decrease significantly, despite our ancestral efforts to defend our highest weight. As you have learned from the stories in this chapter, people who improve their nutrition feel that their bodies are less swollen, their brains are less foggy, they feel more energetic, their joints hurt less, and they enjoy easier movement.

More specifically, I suggest filling the plate with non-starchy, low-glycemic veggies. Such veggies are low in calories and highly satisfying because of their bulk, texture, and fiber. The vegetables combined with adequate protein from plants, fish, and grass-fed animals, and fats from plants, help us feel sated and satisfied. And, if need be, during Sunday Italian family dinners, I recommend using the carbohydrate we crave, such as pasta, as a condiment. For example, place a few strands of pasta on the salad or vegetable-rich meal that is the main component of the meal. This is like adding shredded cheese to a meal. You can still have that savory experience you desire while helping yourself to less of it.

I also invite patients to consider interval or intermittent fasting. Interval fasting involves not eating for extended periods of the day and between meals. Individuals who adopt intermittent fasting go from 12 to 16 hours a day without food or snacks and enjoy meals in the remaining hours. Routinely engaging in interval fasting causes glucose and insulin levels to decline within 2 to 3 months, even if they have been high for years. During the periods when one is not eating, low insulin and glucose allow the liver to deplete its storage of glucose and use fat cells to make energy. Using the fat in your body as an energy source can transform your body into a thinner and younger version of itself.

My husband, Dr. Eric, and I have engaged in a type of interval fasting for decades; we enjoy one meal a day at dinner time. This initially began because we were too busy to eat. Then I discovered that when I did eat lunch, I felt sleepy. We have missed about 40 years of lunches. We have not felt hungry or lost our ability to concentrate. We, in fact, feel more focused and energized. My husband conducts successful surgeries, replacing people's shoulders, hips, and knees during his workday. I support patients all day with my presence, knowledge and heart. For decades, we have maintained normal and stable body weights for our respective heights.

I recommend a more intense form of intermittent fasting to individuals who are obese with a BMI greater than 35. I suggest fasting two days a week, for example, Tuesdays and Fridays or Wednesdays and Saturdays. Individuals who fast two days a week experience greater weight loss. On the two fasting days, individuals keep busy to distract themselves from thinking about food. They limit their calorie intake to between 500 to 600 calories per day, which is reached by drinking broth, water, coffee and tea. Some individuals choose commercially available fast-mimicking programs that can aid in fasting up to five days in a row. Whether personally designed or commercial, the ultimate goal is to improve health by decreasing inflammation through weight reduction.

The most effective method I find to help very high-weight patients lose weight on their own and keep it off is cycling periods of fasting and periods of great healthy whole food. Fasting can be very rewarding at the mind-body-spirit level. I find one's attitude matters. Viewing this method of eating as a gift for the body to be well rather than as painful deprivation or punishment changes the experience.

Fasting can be a bit of a daunting concept. Many of us eat three meals and one to three snacks a day. I recommend easing towards fasting. Begin by slowly decreasing the number of snacks per day. Over a few months, eliminate snacks and one less meal per day. Then attempt to fast for just a single day. Rest assured that the liver will keep us alive. If you plan to try intermittent fasting and have Type II diabetes, talk to your doctor to help you lower your insulin or other glucose-lowering medications as you decrease your carbohydrates and meal frequency. During full fasting days, even if using a fast-mimicking program, I recommend that my patients with Type II diabetes either not take or cut in half their dose of metformin, and, if on insulin, to discuss with me if and how to use insulin during fasting.

Fasting, incredibly renewing for the body, slows your biological-aging clock. While fasting, the body rids itself of toxicities and discards or reuses old and inflamed cells. Fasting decreases inflammation and oxidative stress, promotes weight loss from fat rather than from muscle, and gives the body a chance to improve the health of its DNA.

If you are unwilling or unable to fast, try eating two meals a day and eliminating sugar and processed food. If that is too difficult, keep all your meals but use a smaller plate for each meal. Practice not eating after dinner. I rarely recommend grazing—eating multiple small meals per day—unless eaten within an eight-to-ten-hour period followed by a period of not eating, an interval fast.

We can remember that our ancestral mind-body system resists the discomfort of change. Some discomfort is required to change and retrain our brain to develop new habits and lose weight. If we are willing to go through the struggle to change, we can forge through and recognize that setbacks and discomfort are part of the journey to bring our cells and body back to wellness. The internal fight between the ancestral setpoints and your new consciousness is a normal part of the journey and requires patience and time. We need to cultivate resilience to consistently challenge the fears of our pesky ancestral brains.

How to Sustain Weight Loss

There are additional key elements to losing weight sustainably, regardless of where the weight is located in your body. First, we can take ownership of the process. We can demonstrate that we care for ourselves by continually reminding ourselves of the value of health transformation in our personal lives. We can decide to engage in a weight loss program to improve our lives, not to please our doctor or family, or prepare for an upcoming event that, when it passes, may decrease our motivation to continue the quest for the long term. We can choose to leave a lasting legacy with the transformational choices we make.

Second, gently and consistently improve the quality and decrease the quantity of the foods you ingest. Shop the periphery of the grocery store and skip the aisles which contain shelves of factory-made processed foods. Eat more fruits and vegetables and foods grown in a garden or from the farm.

Third, increase your level of activity or energy expenditure. Two powerful ways to expend more energy are to exercise and decrease insulin to increase fat burning. The best exercise is the exercise we like to do. We can choose to engage in activities we enjoy, such as dancing, hiking, bowling, walking, and yoga. We can join a gym or follow a YouTube workout. Purchasing an activity-tracking device to document the process may help motivate us.

Fourth, we can develop flexibility and patience, especially since none of us are perfectly consistent. This is not an all-or-nothing process. We can feel proud and have confidence that we will succeed in our weight-loss and health-recovery journey if we are consistent 80 percent of the time.

Fifth, we can cultivate compassion for ourselves and develop resiliency, especially since we are now aware of the ancestral mind-body adaptations that contribute to setbacks. We can examine our thoughts and attitude and reframe old mindsets that don't serve us. We can avoid magnifying a setback with negativity or self-derogatory comments and instead become curious about what led to the setback.

Finally, we do not have to be fanatical. Adopting a healthy lifestyle means living a full life. If you are in a French bakery, enjoy a croissant. If it's your birthday, go out for dinner and have dessert. Observe the holidays with your family and friends and enjoy eating what you want. Balance is about giving some leeway to ourselves and striving 80-90 percent of the time to follow a healthy living plan. Showing up every day to do something (even small steps) towards our health goals and self-care matters. We can gently retrain our brains and develop healthy habits. And we can find joy in the process. More and more of us are choosing a sustainable lifestyle and pattern of eating that allows us to enjoy life and savor the food we are eating and sharing with others we love.

My Loving-Kindness Wish for You

May you find comfort being in your body
May you honor your fat cells which have served
you and prior generations so well
May you be released from the brain's old ancestral hold
May your fat cells serve to give you the energy
and protection you need to be well.

Meditation to Enhance Your Journaling

Please scan the QR Code with your Smartphone
or follow this link: https://youtu.be/_SgD_PRe0iQ

Journaling for Transformation

- How did you get to your current health/weight? Are you happy with your current health/weight?
- Have you tried a diet program that has worked for you? What was it and why did it work for you then?

- If you regained weight you had lost, what were the circumstances? What has not worked? Why not?
- If you are overweight or obese, what do you think are the various factors contributing to your weight gain or inability to lose weight, especially after reading this chapter?
- Have you experienced food scarcity or financial issues that affected your diet when you were growing up? Does this affect how you think about food now?
- How is carrying excess weight a response to trauma or an attempt to protect yourself from harm in any way?
- Are cravings an issue for you? Did you know cravings last a short time? You can distract yourself from them or simply ignore them. Cravings increase if (1) we routinely eat refined sugars, high fructose corn syrup, and processed foods; (2) we have lost weight; and (3) we are emotional or stressed out.
- Now that you understand the physical and emotional sources of cravings, how are you preparing to deal with them in a healthy and compassionate way?
- How many meals a day are you having? Can you decrease the number of snacks you are having or the number of meals?
- Now that you know so much, what plan can you create for yourself for attaining a dietary program that you enjoy and that helps to keep you at a healthy weight?
- How can you increase how much you move every day? Have you considered using a monitoring gadget like a step-tracker, Apple watch, Whoop or Oura ring to monitor your movement?
- Other than ancestral mind-body adaptations and habits, do you think you may have a condition that makes it difficult to lose and sustain weight loss? Have you talked to your doctor about this? Perhaps some hormone testing or pharmacologic intervention is indicated in your particular case.

Extra credit: Explain to yourself, or someone else, how we can utilize fat cells to our advantage to lose weight and age more slowly.

Chapter 7

Life Saving Practices

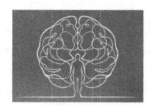

Why Do Some of Us Age Faster?

For millennia the planets have rotated around our sun. The sun rises and sets each day, and the moon goes through its monthly orbit around the earth, causing the earth's ocean tides. Humans have evolved to sleep at night and move during the day in response to these cycles. Humans grow and become fertile at adolescence. Menstrual periods follow a lunar cycle. Humans rear their young up to an age when they reproduce and pass on the family genes to the next generation. After this, there is no evolutionary advantage for the body's biological systems to remain vibrant and alive. There is no advantage for our bodies to retain physical attractiveness or sexuality, structural strength and mobility, memory, or clarity of mind—all the attributes that define a vigorously youthful self-identity.

As we age, hormones decline and negatively impact the state of wellness of the entire body. How we interpret the world and metabolize nutrition are also changed. The body and mind lose internal support systems that keep synaptic connections in the brain intact, sleep gets disturbed, more toxicities accumulate, energy requirements decrease, we actually move less, and insulin resistance increases. Even though the amount of food we eat and our daily movement have not changed, we enter a state of overnutrition When this overnutrition happens, fat accumulates in the abdomen and around internal organs, and body composition changes. The changes in fat deposition and metabolism are inflammatory resulting in less protection for our DNA, cells, muscles, and brain. Muscle mass declines and puts us at higher risk of falling and fracturing bones.

What factors do we need to consider to remain biologically younger for longer as we become chronologically older? Why do some of us age differently than others? These are questions we might ponder after attending a high school reunion. At such gatherings, we see that some of our friends look older and some younger, even though we all share the same chronologic age. When observing our classmates, chronological age—our precise age based on when we were born—does not necessarily correlate with biological age—the inner sense of aliveness and youthfulness that the body energetically expresses. Our friends show variations of biological aging because we all experience different life stressors, diets, and lifestyles. The fact is that the choices we make and how we live our lives make the biggest differences in terms of our aging.

My Story

My mother's mother, abuela Celita, lived until the age of 101. She was using her stationary bike until a month before her death. My mother died before her 90th birthday. She suffered the progressive and devastating consequences of Alzheimer's disease for more than a decade before her death. Alzheimer's is the most common type of dementia. Individuals with dementia show signs of memory loss, impaired reasoning and even personality changes. The symptoms we associate with dementia become increasingly worse over time. Why was my mother so different from her mom? Would this also be my fate?

My mother was a vibrant and beautiful woman who immigrated to the US from Cuba, via Spain, with my dad and four small kids. She had little emotional support through these major transitions. She commuted long distances to her work for years, initially working as a microbiologist and then, after earning a new degree, as a pharmacist. As an immigrant woman, she had significant hurdles to overcome, emotional stresses to cope with, and the worries of a mother with four children in a new country. She did not exercise. She was chronically sleep-deprived, often staying up late and being the first one up to get us all going. She would do anything she was asked if it would help another person be better.

My mother was fully engaged in all aspects of her life until things began to happen. First, she forgot where she parked the car; then she forgot to cook the turkey for the yearly Thanksgiving gathering at her home; she stopped participating in conversations or responding to others; then she forgot where the knobs were in the shower. Her gait became unstable. She even forgot my name. On one of my birthdays, I thanked her for being my mother. She laughed and told me she had never had children, but if she had and I had been her child, she would have liked it very much. She struggled with communication because the wrong words would come out. She lost the capacity to care for and feed herself. I know she remained and lived longer than expected because she was adored by my father, who lovingly tended to, fed, and cared for her along with our dear caretaking team, Ana, Frances, and the rest of us, in my parent's home. This dedicated care continued until the end when she lost the capacity to swallow and left this earth three days later. She and my father held hands at bedtime every night, including the last night. Her illness caused deep sadness for all of us, particularly since we could not help her and the medicines available did not work (as is still the case in 2023).

For the many of us who have observed a loved one decline from Alzheimer's and dementia, we may wonder how we can prevent these diseases from occurring to us. Even though I do not carry the AP04 gene, which increases the risk of developing Alzheimer's earlier in life, I have dedicated a significant amount of time to research. I have learned as much as possible about the causes of Alzheimer's disease and what I can do to reduce my risk for cognitive decline.

As mentioned in a previous chapter, my mom developed inflammatory bowel disease in her forties. After reading Dr. Dale Bredesen's book, *The End of Alzheimer's*, I understood that inflammation in the body from any source can also lead to brain inflammation. Thus, my mother's chronic and ongoing bowel inflammation, along with other factors, may have tipped her over to Alzheimer's disease. This amazing book came out too late to help my mother, but it has given me tools to evaluate the state of my own health and inspired me to get certified in Age Management Medicine. I now understand that Alzheimer's disease is a multifactorial disease with the common threads of inflammation, lack of supportive hormones and other factors that keep nerve connections healthy, and exposure to environmental toxins. No one pill can address this disease. Prevention of this disease requires a multi-system approach with the goal of maintaining healthy brain capacities.

The brain is highly impacted by inflammation and oxidative stress, both being major contributing factors to Alzheimer's disease and vascular dementia. The process of cognitive loss is complex and affected by numerous factors, including but not limited to lifestyle, hormone loss, lack of sleep, head trauma, obesity, diabetes, inflammatory mouth, joint and bowel diseases, virus-induced inflammation, smoking, environmental toxins, alcohol, psychological and emotional stress, too little or too much exercise, and a processed-food, high-sugar diet. The good news is we can make lifestyle choices that reduce the damage caused by these factors and thus support our overall wellness and brain health.

Let's dive in and explore how appropriate lifestyle choices can delay or diminish ancestrally-programmed aging patterns and the risk of brain inflammation. We will consider how we can maintain our vitality and health rather than nurse ill health (as my poor mother did) until we die. Let's learn about the importance of our circadian rhythms and commit to a healthy sleeping and exercise schedule.

Telomeres

Our diet, life stressors, relationships with others, and lifestyle all affect the amount of telomerase we have and the length of our telomeres. As we become older chronologically, telomerase declines, and telomeres shorten naturally. And in some ways, the length of our telomeres defines the biological age we experience. The shorter our telomeres, the higher our risk of dying earlier.

So, what are telomeres?

Chromosomes carry our genetic code through our DNA found inside the nucleus of a cell. Telomeres are the end caps of your chromosomes and function like the aglets at the ends of a shoelace that keep it from fraying. Telomeres protect our chromosomes from damage and maintain the integrity of our individual complex genetic code when our cells divide.

Elizabeth Blackburn won the Nobel Prize because she identified telomerase. Telomerase is an important enzyme that keeps our chromosomes healthy by maintaining the length of our telomeres while our cells divide. Without telomerase, telomeres get shorter; when this happens, the risk of errors during the DNA copying process increases. Once a cell no longer has an accurate copy of DNA, it stops functioning well. These older cells are called senescent cells or "zombie" cells. They are alive but no longer working optimally in the body. These zombie cells cause local inflammation by releasing chemicals that the body does not need and cause oxidative stress. This increases the likelihood of disease, accelerated aging, and premature death.

In Dr. Blackburn's evidence-based and revolutionary book, *The Telomere Effect*, she discusses how shortened telomeres are associated with a variety of lifestyle and psychological factors. Shortened telomeres are caused by a variety of factors, such as:

- inadequate sleep
- poor diet
- emotional and physical trauma
- anxiety and depression
- negative social interactions
- feeling diminished, bullied or shamed
- poor stress interpretation and management
- chronic stress due to caring for ill family members

Likewise, Dr. Blackburn shows that we can make daily choices to increase telomerase levels and lengthen our telomeres. Maintaining the length of our telomeres is clearly associated with proactive action, such as:

- exercise and movement
- changing how we view stress
- stress reduction
- adequate sleep
- a whole food diet
- positive relationships

Telomeres are also affected by hormone changes. For example, chronically elevated cortisol, the stress hormone, shortens telomere length as well as increasing the risk of high blood pressure, weight gain, pre-diabetes, depression, and anxiety. While too much of a hormone can damage telomeres, too little of a hormone is also damaging. For example, women lose their estrogen and progesterone after menopause. The decrease of these hormones is associated with significantly shortened telomeres and decreased telomerase activity. The lack of estrogen and impaired sleep at this time of life contributes to telomere shortening. Therefore, women who receive hormone replacement therapy (HRT) have comparatively longer telomere lengths compared to those who don't receive hormone replacement therapy. If we are unable to use hormones after menopause, then it is crucial to protect the brain with excellent lifestyle habits and diet to help keep the body and mind vibrant.

Hormone decline in women is a clear manifestation of ancestrally programmed aging. It's not fair, but this is the ancestral system's design. Throughout human history, there has been evolutionary selective pressure for humans to live long enough that they can successfully rear their offspring until they can survive and reproduce themselves, thus successfully passing their genes to the next generation. Once this ancient biological purpose was accomplished, there was no selective pressure for continuing to maintain normal hormone levels in women. Now humans routinely live well beyond age 40, but our ancient biology did not change despite our recently longer lifespans in the last 100 years. One of the problems we experience is that the lack of hormones like estrogen, progesterone, or testosterone do not just affect telomere length, but also lessens the integrity of established neuronal connections in the brain. Over time this contributes to loss of cognition, among other factors discussed. The good news is that menopausal hormone deficiency can be successfully addressed for most women through using bioidentical hormone replacement therapy, estradiol, and progesterone, started shortly after or within the first six years of menopause. Contraindications for HRT include having breast cancer or a strong family history of this disease. Some genetic mutations, like the breast cancer gene, BRCA, increase breast cancer risk significantly. For additional information, check out my YouTube videos, "Bioidentical Hormones: What are They? Should I have Them?" https://www.youtube.com/watch?v=vo1RZ5mUq9Q and "Menopause Transition Masterclass https://youtu.be/XD0JnGARXpI. For additional information see the Resource section of this book.

Sirtuins

Just as important as our mitochondria and telomeres are the sirtuins. *Sirtuins* are highly conserved proteins. They are found across numerous species, from yeast to humans. Sirtuins work in the nucleus to protect our cell's DNA replication, repair, and appropriate cell death (apoptosis). They prevent premature telomere attrition. Sirtuins work in our mitochondria to facilitate the energy-making process using NAD, manage oxidative stress and inflammation, and regulate carbohydrate metabolism. These proteins are vital. However, poor food choices, too much insulin, all sources of inflammation, inactivity, etc., all interfere with the function of these essential proteins. As a result, they are unable to do their work in protecting our DNA from damage or help in making energy. This results in faster aging because dead cells, or zombie cells, hang out for longer and cause inflammation around them. Damaged DNA increases the risk of cancers, rapid aging, and metabolic havoc. Fortunately, we can do a lot about this. Eating whole foods, increasing the amount of plants and fruits in our diet, and considering decreasing or letting go of red meats and dairy. Fewer meals a day or more fasting helps. Lowering sugar intake and insulin response is huge to really help you age well. Consider taking supplements that help sirtuins work better, like resveratrol and quercetin. Also, allow the body the lifestyle it ancestrally requires for healing and longevity to occur. Talk to your doctor about taking metformin. Ask about tests to see how you are aging so you are better informed about gauging your aging process. I recommend reading Dr. David Sinclair's book *Lifespan*. I don't know him yet, and I am not getting paid by him, but his science is solid. To make your body heartier, allow yourself to feel a little hungry, move fast enough to make yourself a little out of breath most days. If the season allows, get some exposure to cold air. These experiences tell your body that it's time to be resilient, younger, and ready for a long and healthy future.

Our Circadian Rhythm Matters

The circadian rhythm is the natural cycle of changes the body goes through in a 24-hour period. These changes are physical, mental and behavioral. Every single cell in our body has an internal biological clock that aligns with our day-night, wake-sleep cycles and regulates most hormonal and metabolic events that occur in the body. If you mess around with your natural circadian rhythms, you suffer.

The circadian clock is primarily regulated by light at the start of the day and then the increasing dark of the night. If you have a routine schedule in which you wake up and go to sleep at a certain time each day and have your meals at a regular time, then your circadian clock and you are in sync. Without a routine, our circadian rhythm is not in sync. As a result, our metabolism slows down, and we suffer from more illness and disease.

What happens to our physiology when the sun rises each morning? The light is sensed by the retina, a membrane that lines the back of the inside of our eye. The retina converts light, form, and color into chemical neural energy and sends signals to the hypothalamus, a structure inside the middle of the head near the pituitary gland that regulates our hormones. These signals reach the hypothalamus's suprachiasmatic nucleus and trigger a neurochemical signal to our pituitary, adrenal and other organs. These signals wake us up and facilitate the secretion of the morning hormones that signal the liver to get ready to digest and metabolize the foods that will soon come.

There are daytime hormones and nighttime hormones. For example, testosterone and cortisol levels are highest in the morning. Both hormones decline in the evening. The approximate 12 hours of daylight is the circadian time when digestion and metabolism of nutrients are best. Eating late or in the middle of the night is not part of ancestral programming.

As light declines in the evening, the retina lets the pineal gland know that it is time to start to rest. The pineal gland is an important part of the endocrine system that regulates circadian rhythms by releasing melatonin. The pineal gland releases more melatonin when it is dark and less when it is light. Melatonin is a hormone that influences immune function, cortisol levels, and blood pressure. Melatonin also improves sleep. Sleep is the time when repair, restoration, renewal, and detoxification of the mind-body unit, occurs. At night, night hormones, such as growth hormones, get secreted. While sleeping at night, children grow, and our muscles are renewed and repaired. Thyroid-stimulating hormone secretion also happens at night. These hormones control our weight, muscle strength, body temperature, and mood.

While respecting the circadian rhythm is crucial for our hormonal and overall health and well-being, the circadian clock is resistant to change. When we travel to another time zone or shift to daylight saving time, our inner clock struggles to adapt to the change. The brain feels stressed, and our body experiences toxic oxidative stress. This discord with our inner clock results in temporary damaging effects to the body and mind. For example, in the first week after we initiate daylight saving time, there is an increased risk of strokes and heart attacks, more accidents, and major disruptions in quality of life for families with small children. The long-term negative effects associated with these human-scheduled time shifts include increases in heart disease, cancer of the liver, obesity, mood disorders, and substance abuse. Based on the data, the American Association of Sleep Medicine has recommended that we remain on standard time all year.

Protect the Brain with Sleep

A key component to protecting the brain is to guard the quality and quantity of our sleep. When we sleep, we are not conscious and the body is not mobile. Though sleep is a recurring state that allows our nervous system to relax, the processes in the brain and body that keep us alive continue to function.

Sleep supports our body and brain to function well. Most of us need 7 to 9 hours of sleep each night to experience the restorative benefits of sleep. In general, good sleep habits and practices help us maintain alertness and energy, balance our hormones and metabolism, enhance our memory and abilities to concentrate, and create longer telomeres.

Our learning and creativity are enhanced. We are better able to manage our emotions and handle stress. Sleep keeps us healthier and reduces our risk for disease.

Recently, researchers have discovered that the brain opens up a drainage system while we are sleeping. This drainage system is called the *glymphatic system*, and it rids our brain of toxic waste substances that we have created in our neural networks during the day. Thinking and stress processing occurs through chemical reactions in our brain. For example, amyloid, a protein that accumulates in the nerve cells of people who have Alzheimer's disease, actively gets cleared out of neurons during sleep while the glymphatic drainage system is open.

There is an actual structure to our sleep. During the night, the brain transitions through different electro-chemical sleep stages: light, deep, and REM (rapid eye movement). Each of these cycles occurs about every 90 minutes. Light sleep takes up most of our sleep time. We can easily be awakened during this time. From light sleep, we enter into deep sleep. During deep sleep, which typically happens most during the first half of our sleeping period, both the mind and body are repaired, renewed, and detoxified. Cell regeneration, tissue repair, and growth occur. Our immune function is strengthened. During this stage, the body is deeply relaxed, and it is difficult for the sleeper to be awakened. Aerobic exercise during the day and going to bed at the right time will increase the duration of deep sleep. During REM sleep, we experience rapid eye movements and dream more. Dreams allow us to synthesize our day-to-day experiences. Though our eyes are moving more rapidly, we're actually paralyzed during this stage of sleep, which is helpful because it keeps us from acting out our dreams or kicking our partners. During REM sleep, we process and integrate daily events and learning into memory for future use. These different sleep cycles—light sleep, deep sleep, and REM sleep—alternate throughout the night.

On waking, one of the most helpful things we can do is to experience sunlight or bright light for at least 15 to 30 minutes. When sunlight enters the eyes and retina, the entire brain lights up. Research substantiates that early morning light helps us sleep better at night. During the winter in cold climates, if there are no windows and gray skies persist, light therapy has been shown to help individuals with Seasonal Affective Disorder (SAD). Some of these lights are even branded as "happy lights," as light is known to elevate our mood. I urge my patients affected by SAD to use SAD lights for 15 to 30 minutes each morning to maintain the circadian rhythm.

During the day, we can develop habits to improve our chances of a good night's sleep. We can stick to a schedule and routine, eat healthily, avoid too much caffeine, include physical activity, manage stress, and avoid napping during the day. We can also stop eating early in the evening so that we are not fueling ourselves just before trying to sleep.

More and more people suffer from disorders that interfere with the quality of their sleep. Snoring and sleep apnea are common disorders. Snoring is vibrational noise in the airway. Apnea is more serious. The vibrational airway noise is present, but so is a pause in our breathing. The starts and stops to breathing, lead to nightmares and multiple nighttime awakenings, which damages the cycles of sleep. As a result, those with sleep apnea wake feeling unrested, tend to fall asleep during the day and often feel hungrier.

Sleep disorders, such as sleep apnea, impact our hormones. When we don't sleep well, more ghrelin, the hunger hormone, is released by the stomach, so we feel hungrier during the day. Women experience a change of hormones at menopause that also contributes to sleep disturbances leading to feeling hungrier during the day. Relief can be provided with either hormone replacement or with non-hormonal methods.

Most common to those with sleep apnea is the release of stress hormones activated by the fight or flight survival system. During periods when we are not breathing during sleep, the body reacts as if it were suffocating because it's not getting enough oxygen. When the body-mind unit senses this life-threatening stress, the sympathetic-stress management system is activated, and adrenaline and cortisol are secreted into the bloodstream all night. If sleep apnea happens regularly, the heart rate and blood pressure go up. This is a chronic stress that will negatively affect telomere length. Fortunately, sleep apnea can be successfully treated.

Furthermore, lack of sleep damages and prematurely ages the brain by decreasing our capacity to protect our neurons and increasing the risk of developing cognitive decline, dementia, and Alzheimer's disease. Although we can become weak if we go days without eating or drinking, we can't go without sleeping for an extended period of time without experiencing harmful effects. In fact, sleep is *so* ancestrally defended that if our brain senses a major deficit, we will fall asleep at places we don't expect or intend, like in the car while driving.

So, what can we do to maximize our chances of getting good sleep? Experts have coined the term "sleep hygiene" to help us develop better bedtime habits to sleep well. We can make the following proactive choices to improve our sleep hygiene:

- Make the bedroom and bed inviting.
- Decrease the bedroom temperature.
- Eliminate gadgets that light up, beep, or flash.
- Create a quiet and dark space.
- Prior to going to sleep, use lighting that is warm, soft, and soothing, and avoid blue light, such as from an iPad, computer, or smartphone.
- Stretching before bedtime, doing gentle yoga (yoga nidra), journaling, and focusing on our breath can make a difference by resetting the state of the brain to allow us to fall asleep.

All of these choices help you fall asleep faster. Consider making your bed a sacred place where you only make love and sleep. If you eat, write, watch television, or work from your bed, the brain gets confused about what should happen in bed.

I have been tracking the quality of my sleep for the past 2-3 years. This self-monitoring has helped me figure out how to maximize the quality of my sleep and detect the factors that interfere with it. I obtain better restorative sleep and keep my body healthier when I practice certain habits. These positive habits include getting to bed early and at the same time, exercising during the day, not eating 2-3 hours before I go to sleep, avoiding alcoholic drinks, avoiding news and difficult conversations late in the evening, and creating a sleep-supportive environment.

Many patients ask me what supplements are helpful for sleep in addition to creating excellent sleep hygiene habits. I have tried various types of preparations to help myself and my patients. I do not get paid by any company for offering these suggestions. I have found that melatonin is helpful for falling asleep but not to sustain it unless you use a slow-release preparation. Melatonin tablets need to be taken one hour before bedtime. Melatonin liquid works faster, and a dosage of 3 mg or less is very effective. The ideal dose for any individual can vary between one to ten milligrams. You can feel groggy in the morning if you take too high a dosage. I learned from the Ayurvedic medicine tradition that hot milk with cardamom and ginger is very soporific before bedtime. To calm the nervous system, I like L-theanine 100 mg and/or magnesium citrate or glycinate 100 to 200 mg at bedtime. Avoid magnesium if you have chronic kidney disease. I like SleepyTime Extra by Celestial Seasonings, which has chamomile and valerian. Women in menopause who cannot take hormone replacement can use medications like gabapentin to calm the nervous system and decrease hot flashes, which tend to wake women up. I do not prescribe sleep medicines or benzodiazepines ever, as these can become addictive and interfere with the quality of your sleep. Lastly, it's important to know that when we are depressed or have some other physical illness, sleep can be impaired. It is a good idea to have your primary care doctor evaluate you and assess if some other treatment is needed.

Case Study: JP's Story

One of my female patients, JP, a 65-year-old executive, came to see me because she was suffering from severe insomnia. I shared with her something I offer many of my patients with sleep disorders. I suggested that she consider treating herself as she would her own child or grandchild. She would naturally want this child to grow and thrive and would understand that a child benefits from going to bed at a fixed time every night. She would make sure that the child was comfortable and undisturbed while sleeping. She is also worthy of the same care with her own sleep experience.

JP was intrigued by the idea that she could train herself to sleep better by treating herself as she does her grandchild. She took the challenge. She earnestly had herself go to sleep and wake up at the same time for three weeks, and she applied all the sleep hygiene suggestions. She expressed her amazement at the follow-up appointment that this simple method actually worked and said, "Who knew? I can now sleep like a baby." The results? She feels more energetic and effective in both her personal and professional life.

Over the years, I have observed and experienced that we can all train our brain, even if we are currently struggling with sleep problems and disorders, to sleep better. In summary, our sleep is enhanced by having consistent good habits. Following a fixed wake and sleep schedule, using morning sun or light therapy in the morning, adding a little melatonin at night, prioritizing our sleep hygiene and making proactive choices that demonstrate we care enough about ourselves.

Exercise Heals & Transforms

"I've been exercising, but I'm not losing weight." This is a comment that I hear from many of my patients. Losing weight does not occur from exercise alone. However, when we exercise we send signals to the rest of the body that help our metabolism and our brain's appetite perception work better. Exercise also makes us more resilient to the negative effects of poor diet and stress. The body is wise about conserving energy so it can also adapt its metabolism based on energy expenditures. For example, ultramarathoners who regularly train, decrease the calories they use over time. For those of us trying to lose weight, improving our diet is critical in order to maintain our muscle mass while we lose our fat mass. The combination of exercise with whole-food nutrition, good sleep and lower stress are essential for the body to normalize hormones and let go of the excess weight. While exercise should be done at the time that is best for each of us, some studies suggest that doing it at different times may help different people. For weight-loss, doing exercise while fasting is more effective, whereas afternoon exercise is better if you are dealing with a metabolic problem like diabetes. If you are building muscle and a normal weight, then fasting before exercise does not make sense and having protein before and after exercise would be prudent.

Exercise is movement that requires physical effort and enhances our well-being. When we exercise, we are communicating to our body and mind that our physical presence and strength matters, and it's not time for aging. I like for my exercise to be fun and functional for my needs. My three personal goals are to be able to run 2-3 miles at any time, just in case of an emergency, dance 1-2 hours at a party, and be able to lift a 30-pound suitcase into the overhead compartment of an airplane.

All conventional medical societies recommend at least 30 minutes of exercise every day. What kind of exercise is best? I suggest choosing movement that brings you joy and to consider an intensity of movement that is moderate. Moderate exercise means that we are moving at such an intensity that we are a little bit short of breath, though we can keep a conversation going. When we engage in moderate exercise, we are using more oxygen as energy and improving our fitness.

Fitness is a combined expression of our strength, endurance, and aerobic capacity. Strength is the ability to provide force against resistance. Endurance is the power to sustain physical activity. Aerobic capacity (VO2max) is a measurement of our maximal ability to use oxygen during vigorous exercise. The higher our VO2max, the more fit we are and the lower our risk of prematurely dying.

We have learned that longer telomeres are important for our health and longevity. There are two types of exercise that promote longer telomeres and keep us fit. Aerobic exercise, which includes any activity which gets our heart and lungs working hard and makes us sweat, such as fast walks, dancing, running, jogging, tennis, biking, and climbing stairs, are all helpful. The second exercise type is high-intensity interval training (HIIT), a program alternating periods of moderate and higher exercise intensity during a 20 to 30-minute period of time. HIIT produces healthy physical stress on the body as your heart rate increases and decreases. These exercises stimulate the increase of hormones from fat cells and other sites to reduce blood sugar, help insulin work better, and increase our oxygen consumption to keep our energy expenditure demands high. Engaging in HIIT three times a week is an efficient use of your valuable time and helps your telomeres remain long. It is healthy to be active enough to make yourself a little out of breath at some point every day.

While aerobic exercise is essential, I also recommend movement that supports us to maintain flexibility and tend to our posture. Flexibility can be maintained with regular stretching routines and yoga. Yoga, once or twice a week, increases our flexibility and improves additional aspects of our mind-body wellness, including posture. Most of us use computers and phones for hours each day, which forces our heads forward and causes a hunched-over posture. The effects of this change in our posture are numerous—headaches, neck problems, and pain in our upper shoulders and spine. My husband, an orthopedic surgeon, frequently sees patients with posture problems in his practice. He recommends trying to keep our head balanced over our pelvis, not slouched in front. Numerous gadgets exist that remind us to stand up or straighten up when we lean forward. These may be worth purchasing if we have trouble reminding ourselves to hold our heads back and aligned with our spine.

Strength training is a vital form of exercise that can support us with a challenging aspect of aging—losing muscle mass. Ancestrally, as we start to age, we experience sarcopenia, an age-related loss of muscle mass. Sarcopenia is caused by moving less and the decline of muscle-supporting hormones, such as DHEA, testosterone and growth hormone. People with low muscle mass and fitness levels are more prone to fall and fracture their bones. Strength training with weights or resistance bands can reduce our risk of such falls and fractures. Pilates is also a great form of core and strength training. Tai Chi, ballet, bar exercises, and yoga help to improve our balance.

The benefits of exercise are abundant. When we choose to move our bodies and exercise, we experience less depression, less anxiety and less inflammation or joint pains. Remember that inflammation is the root of most diseases and premature death. Exercise is an anti-inflammatory treatment. Proper exercise improves your metabolism and can even prevent damage caused by less healthy foods since exercise helps your liver to metabolize foods better. Exercise strengthens your bones and muscles, increases the blood flow to the brain, and for many people, is just as effective as taking an antidepressant. When we choose to exercise, we are giving ourselves the gift of having a younger biological age and reducing our risk for age-related diseases. One of the most powerful and effective prescriptions I offer you is the prescription of exercise.

My Loving-Kindness Wish for You

May you feel rested upon awakening
May you feel physically fit and strong
May you embrace the wisdom of your internal clock.

Meditation to Enhance Your Journaling

Please scan the QR Code with your Smartphone
or follow this link: https://youtu.be/dP3LtZmgAqU

Journaling for Transformation

1. **Sleep**
   - Do you wake up rested?
   - How many hours do you sleep?
   - Do you go to bed when you feel tired?
   - What is your routine for going to sleep?
   - What makes your bedroom a comfortable place to sleep?
   - How many gadgets are in your room (TV, phones, computers, etc.)?
   - Are you using your computer or cell phone until bedtime?
   - How many people sleep with you? How many pets? Do they wake you up?
   - Do you snore? Has your partner gone to sleep in another room?
   - Can you commit to waking up and going to sleep at the same time every day for 30 days?
   - We evolved to respond to lightness and dark, what steps can you take to tend better your internal clock?

2. **Exercise**

   Plan and schedule regular times to exercise and ink these times on your calendar. Respect yourself by showing up. Making exercise fun and playful can help you exercise routinely. Persistence and consistency matter in creating a new habit.

   - What is your favorite way to exercise?
   - How often do you really exercise?
   - Do you enjoy exercise while doing it?
   - Can you make your exercise or movement experience more fun? (Listening to music or good lectures or doing it with a friend).
   - Given what you now know, could you explain to a friend why exercise would help them?

Care of The Soul

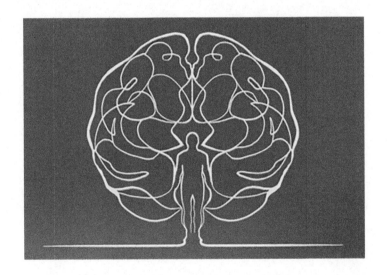

Chapter 8

The Outer Family, Friends & Culture

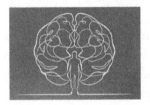

Navigating Obstacles

Obstacles and setbacks are an inevitable part of the change-making process. While some of the obstacles and setbacks may arise from within, external forces also influence our journey to healthier living. Many common challenges relate to how others react when they see us change for the better. Other challenges come from social situations or environments that created or nurtured behaviors and mindsets we are now trying to change, called social conditioning. We need awareness and special skills to navigate these challenging spaces. Sometimes it is difficult for family and friends to accept the adjustments we are making to create change. We may even be guilty of doing the same when we see a loved one change. Why is it hard to recognize that it is normal and healthy for all of us to grow and change?

Unfortunately, many of us have fixed expectations and ideas about one another and our behaviors. By now, you know that our ancestral brain feels safe when things are known, predictable, and static. Adopting a growth mindset is one of the key skills that we and others can develop to increase flexibility and support the personal growth of ourselves and others. Such a mindset increases our capacity to communicate with authenticity and extend love and compassion for ourselves and each other. A growth mindset can help us see each other as evolving people rather than as people stuck in fixed roles.

My Story

When I became engaged to Eric, his paternal grandparents, who have since passed, were dismayed that their first grandson was planning his life with a Cuban woman. Without ever meeting me, they warned him that he would never become a "society doctor" if he was associated with me. They withdrew all invitations and opportunities they had originally extended to us as a newly engaged couple *before* they learned I was Cuban Latina. There were no further discussions, and they did not attend our wedding. I had never faced such intensely targeted and personalized discrimination and was deeply saddened by that experience of rejection. At the time, I was too young and did not have the skills to process this devastating awareness that someone felt I was not good enough, did not belong, and that I was not worthy. Thankfully, the essence of my being was aroused and activated! I could lift up my head, stand up and be proud that I was my parents' daughter and a good and smart person. Despite their reaction, we forged on and continue to be happily married and serve with integrity as professionals in our community decades later.

As I write this, I can feel that that younger part of me is still sad about this. Thinking about this time causes a small ache in my throat and heart, where my body has kept score. So, the mature, wise adult I am now tends to the hurt, younger part of me, reminding her that she belongs and she was always good and whole. I tell her that those people had limited capacity to grow and lacked the wisdom to see her essence or to act differently. I explain to the younger me that they were racists and because they were, they lost a chance for more love and connection.

How can we overcome hurdles and enrich our relationships with ourselves and others as we grow and change? How can we remain whole through the process and uphold our visions for wellness? How can we make changes to improve our life and inspire others to join us?

The Value of Generative Conversations

Earlier, we explored transformation, our mind and the inner family system—especially the younger parts and learned ways to create more inner balance within our mind-body system. Here we will learn to enhance our skills in communicating with others. Proficiency in these skills empowers us to forge successful change and communicate our needs and intentions in ways that engage others to support us. One of the most powerful ways to seek and obtain the support of others is to engage in *generative conversations.*

Conversations are an important part of every human relationship— relationships with ourselves, family, friends, colleagues, neighbors and even strangers. Conversations can connect or disconnect us. Learning how to have a conversation that expands beyond politeness and doesn't disintegrate into misunderstandings and division can foster deeper connections and serve our individual and social health.

Generative conversations are a particular kind of conversation than can give life to and energize our relationships. I learned about this type of conversation from Dr. Claire Zammit, founder of the Institute for Feminine Power, Evolving Wisdom, and The Institute for Women-Centered Coaching, Training and Leadership. She is one of my brilliant mentors whose influence has benefited both my personal and work life.

Engaging in a generative conversation means becoming clear on what we as an adult need and want to let another, or others, know. The goal of a generative conversation is that both sides gain insight, grow from the experience, develop trust and leave with a better understanding of each other.

All vital conversations can benefit from some preparation. Since the younger and unhealed parts of ourselves can be triggered when we engage in more important and challenging conversations, we must take some time beforehand to ground and center into our wise-adult self. A slow-breath meditation can decrease the likelihood of more confrontational, insecure, hurt or grieved parts showing up and taking over the conversation. When the driver of the conversation is a younger and more emotionally hurt part of us that feels disenfranchised, unheard, revengeful, angry, or jealous, we may easily activate the other party's ancestral stress system. Then both parties are disconnected from their higher and more rational thought centers. When the fight-flight-freeze system is ignited and individuals engaged in a conversation have lost a sense of safety and trust, the conversation deteriorates. This is why a generative conversation with others or ourselves requires some preparation.

While engaged in this healing conversation, we make an effort, even if it is difficult, to see the other person with positive regard and compassion. We set the intention to embrace their gifts, talents, follies, vulnerabilities, humanity, and to see their wholeness with the aim to understand their point of view, as we hope they will do for us. We are aware that they may have assumptions about us and the changes we are making. We accept that we also possess notions about them and what they know, whether these ideas are right or wrong. The conversation provides an opportunity to ask questions and to correct misconceptions.

When we engage in a generative conversation, we are creating an open space where curiosity, compassion and creativity can coexist. With the intention for a nonjudgmental discussion, we deeply listen to one another and share our perspectives. As a result, erroneous assumptions are disrupted, and mutual feelings of safety and trust increase. A greater understanding of the situation and one another transpires. New possibilities arise to solve problem areas. Growth and empowerment emerge for everyone in such a conversation.

The stories in this chapter will illustrate the value of conversations in which we are trying to accomplish a goal, create greater connectivity, and receive support from others or our internal family system members. These conversations are crucial to overcoming obstacles and sustaining the changes we are making, especially all changes at the level of self-identity in any domain of our life: personal, professional or spiritual.

Obstacles: Misunderstandings, Faulty Assumptions & Resistance

When we begin to make changes, we develop new beliefs and behaviors congruent with the healthy self-identity we are seeking. As we begin to feel better, our confidence increases. Our clothing fits better. We may wear brighter colors and experiment with new styles. Because we are making different choices and behaving in new ways, our family and friends may express discomfort with some of these changes.

Imagine, for example, that our intimate partner, children, friends, or acquaintances are accustomed to how we look, dress, and behave and then we decide to make some changes to our appearance. Perhaps we start wearing tighter jeans with colorful tops. Or we choose a new hairstyle and maybe even hair color. We wear a pair of heels instead of tennis shoes. Sometimes, this kind of change can create discomfort in family members. They may wonder what's going on with us. They may feel nervous. They might prefer how we used to dress and show up and express their dislike over our new appearance.

Catherine, one of my colleagues, remembers such a situation that occurred when she was in middle school. One evening her mother came home wearing white go-go boots. Catherine expressed her horror. What if her friends would see her wearing those crazy go-go boots! What an embarrassment! Catherine accused her of trying to act like a teenager. The magnitude of Catherine's reaction caused her mother to return the boots to the store.

The fear of our parents embarrassing us is common. We don't want our parents behaving in ways contrary to what we expect of them. These expectations may come from cultural and family norms, fearing what others think, or simply from not wanting our parents to change, even if the change is better for them. It takes maturity to recognize that how someone dresses or shows up is an expression of their current and evolving identity and not a reflection of who *we* are.

Case Study: Mary, Louise & Jean's Stories

When we ourselves change physically, others may make assumptions or have inner concerns or reactions regarding how our physical change might affect them personally. Three of my patients, Mary, Louise, and Jean, conveyed how others reacted toward them after they lost significant weight.

Mary, a cancer survivor, lost weight during her treatments for cancer. She appreciated her new lease on life and enjoyed her appearance and lower weight. To continue to support her health, she was eating differently than before her cancer diagnosis. Her husband, however, continued to interpret her lower weight as a sign of illness and of the possibility of losing her companionship, so he continually counteracted her efforts at weight maintenance by bringing her cakes and cookies in order to support his inner belief that he would feel safer if she was a little heavier.

Louise, another patient, described Sam, her partner's, feelings about her weight and appearance makeover. He wondered if something was wrong with Louise. Was she involved in a relationship with somebody else? Was there something amiss between them? Sam became suspicious and controlling.

Jean, the third patient, described the reactions of her coworkers after her pandemic weight loss. Some congratulated her. Some behaved in new passive-aggressive ways. It turned out that several of these coworkers had also been trying to lose weight before the pandemic. The pandemic set them back, and instead of losing, Jean's coworkers gained weight. Likely, they felt frustrated that Jean successfully achieved weight loss and they had not. They acted out their frustration by ignoring or treating her with disdain.

When we are committed to transformation, the individuals who are part of our everyday life often make wrong assumptions about why we are making the changes. They need our help to understand what making these changes mean for us. Otherwise, misunderstandings lead to emotional reactions and behaviors that reflect immaturity and a lack of understanding of a situation. These reactions are not only painful and disconnecting, but can sabotage our efforts to reach our health goals and feel well.

By considering our new understanding of the mind-body connection and the ancestral nervous system response, it's possible to transform misunderstandings that result in disconnection into understanding and connection. Recall that we often perceive change as unsettling and potentially dangerous, especially when such change does not fit our fixed mindset or expectations. This starts our brain scrambling to make logic out of our perceptions, forming thoughts and assumptions, and in turn, triggering our emotions. Emotions activate our ancestral survival system, which is always working to determine whether the situation we are facing is safe or dangerous. Lastly, reactive behaviors emerge to protect or soothe us from the perceived threat.

We must apply ways to calm down our central nervous system and subdue the ancestral survival response. The first step of reflecting on our own complex human nature and tendencies is critical, as is translating what we think into action. A high level of consciousness and vulnerability are needed to disrupt original assumptions through mutual understanding and good communication skills.

Helping Others Accept Our Changes

Mary, my first patient, and I reassured her husband that she was cancer free. I informed him that maintaining a lower weight and exercising has been shown to decrease cancer recurrence. With this increased awareness, Mary's husband joined her, and they both are working together to improve their health. He is now comfortable with Mary's leaner figure.

Louise, my second patient, confided to her partner, Sam, that she had been feeling insecure about her weight. Explaining her excess weight prevented her from being more sexually intimate with him. The desire for a loving and intimate relationship motivated her to lose weight, increase her fitness and feel better about herself. Sam, who initially feared that Louise was emotionally distancing herself, was relieved to understand that the physical change in Louise was a sign that she valued their intimacy. Louise understood why Sam's fear had activated uncharacteristic behaviors and that she was deeply loved by Sam regardless of her weight or appearance. Their willingness to apply generative conversation to the situation resulted in an increased understanding for each other. Their empathy and compassion also rose and markedly improved their relationship.

Jean, the third patient, applied generative conversation skills to her work situation. Jean asked her boss and coworkers if it might be possible to have vegetables and fruits instead of cookies, at the weekly office meeting. When asked why, she was honest, explaining that she was trying to reverse a pre-diabetes diagnosis by making and consistently upholding changes to her lifestyle and food habits. Her vulnerability opened up a group discussion. Other coworkers shared concerns about their health. Everyone agreed that changing the office environment could help the entire office. Jean's openness generated support for herself and her coworkers.

As we can see, opening-up and sharing what is going on invites others to do the same. The usefulness of letting others know our thoughts and feelings about a situation can clear up assumptions and misunderstandings, reveal shared values, provide a space for others to share what is true for them, and ultimately improve relationships.

Managing Our Reactions

When we commit to making changes, we might falsely believe that it's entirely up to us to make these changes. However, we all have the human need to belong and be accepted. So, the feedback we receive from others informs our connection with them and influences our own inner reality. If the feedback is questionable or critical, our ancestral mind-body system is triggered, which can raise our own insecurities and halt us from moving forward to realize a change.

Guess who comes forward and acts up to protect us when we are triggered? If you responded, "our inner family system," you are right. Members of our internal family system ignite a dialogue in our head. Inner comments like the following can deflate our commitment to change:

- May Day! May Day! There's a serious problem here.
- If you keep changing, it's over. They're going to reject you.
- What's going to happen if you keep changing?
- You sure you want to keep on doing this?
- I don't like how this is going.
- Here we go! You are going to be hurt again.

This inner dialogue from our younger internal family system members is to be expected. These younger parts want to protect us from harm and loss of connection to others but in immature and primitive ways. Welcome this dialogue. This kind of inner talk indicates that we are truly changing the ways of the past to align to our current desires and authentic values. Rather than belittle or condemn our inner family system members, we can choose to respond with kindness, compassion, and wisdom to the feedback we receive. Everyone needs reassurance, especially the younger less secure parts of our internal system. Assure these parts that we will survive making these changes and improve our health and well-being, as a result.

Dealing with Our Inner Critic

When we are striving for a new way of being, we must remain particularly aware and lovingly patient with the perfectionist parts of our internal family system. Our inner perfectionists can feel threatened and insecure when we are aiming to create lasting change. If we are unaware of the existence or do not expect perfectionistic parts to emerge, we can be held back from forming our new healthy self-identity. These members of the inner family system are the least flexible and have the most difficulty accepting change. They have developed ways to control everything so they are not criticized and feel safe. They fear humiliation and negative outcomes that they may have felt or experienced from others at a younger age when they could not defend themselves or put what was happening in the right context. They staunchly protect their old primitive behaviors, rituals, and habits that they created to keep us safe. The perfectionist parts criticize and belittle. They imagine and present scenarios that prove we will fail to meet the mark. They are insistent that we listen to them. If they are successful, we may begin to procrastinate and sabotage our efforts, which, in turn, activates more dissatisfaction, self-blame, and shame.

I know the realities and pressures of the inner critic. I have had personal experiences with my fearful inner critic. Most recently, my inner perfectionist made concerted efforts to stunt the writing and completion of this book. I applied the skills discussed throughout the book to calm the fears of this part of me. I took a few minutes to simply breathe. Then I connected with my current age wise-adult to access my inner wisdom. In this calmer wiser condition, I sent love and appreciation to my perfectionistic inner family member. I thanked them for their concern and efforts to protect me from pain, and the real or imagined criticism from others. I reminded my inner critic (as I frequently do) that it is perfectly normal to be imperfect and human. I reassured my inner critic that writing this book from my feminine perspective would make my book more interesting, unique, and helpful to its readers. I subdued my perfectionist inner family member by reminding them that I could handle any criticism that came our way. I had their back. I embraced all of their suffering and loved them no matter what, even when they challenged me with all their perfectionistic worries. Finally, I suggested they go have fun and play.

Learning to behold our imperfections, with acceptance and compassion helps us embrace the process of transformation and enjoy the journey of growth. Two great resources that have served me and thousands of others are two books by Tara Brach, *Radical Acceptance* and *Radical Compassion*. You don't have to meet a person to have them influence your life. Tara is one of my spiritual mentors. I have not yet had the pleasure to meet her and thank her in person for the light she brings to me and others. Her insights helped me grow and navigate dark times.

Asking for Help & Accepting It

Many of us need to develop the essential skills of asking for help *and* accepting help from others. These skills are a sign of shifting from a scarcity mindset to an abundant mindset. My female patients admit that asking for help from others does not come naturally or instinctually to them. Many of my patients have full-time jobs outside the home and state that they do not have time to exercise, meditate or go to sleep on time because they have chores to complete around the house. Interestingly, many of them have a partner or adult children living with them who could help with those chores. But their mindset prevents that from happening. The following are common remarks I have heard over the years:

- My husband and children's jobs are more important than mine, so I can't bother them to do house things.

- If I don't do the housework or cook, my family will feel deprived of my care and love. I would not be a good mother.
- I feel frustrated. No one is helping. They should know better.

The first comment depicts what I have heard many women say over the years. These patients are not valuing themselves, their work, or their needs. Our work is equally important as the work of others and our needs matter. The second comment reveals a fixed mindset around what constitutes a good mother, wife, and homemaker and limits the patient's options. The third comment reveals that this individual is assuming the other family members know what she needs or wants. All of these socially conditioned mindsets and assumptions need to be disrupted so more growth and possibilities can be reached.

Case Study: Maggie's Story

At times, we may act in ways that confirm to our partners or family members that we have everything under control and don't need help when we actually feel overwhelmed. Maggie, one of my patients, used the generative conversation approach to enroll her partner in helping around the house so she could have more self-care time. Entering the conversation and expressing her vulnerability created the safety and trust for her partner to become aware and act on her needs. She confided that she had a difficult time asking for help but realized that she needed to learn. Maggie was surprised at the outcome. Her partner was eager to help, and since their conversation, has taken on more responsibilities to provide additional support. Maggie is slowly learning how to drop the superwoman role and become more comfortable with taking care of herself. She realizes that her mindset limited her and the obstacles she perceived were self-made. More importantly, she and her husband now see each other with more compassion.

Equally as important as developing the capacity to *ask* for support is developing the capacity to *accept* that support. I had the chance to work on developing these skill sets on a recent visit to my daughter and her husband. As a sign of my motherly love, I enjoy cooking for them.

However, during this visit I also had a work deadline. A part of me felt guilty that I had to work during this visit. I thought I was not being a *good* mother if I didn't cook dinner for them. I realized that my perceptions or mindset about my role as a mother created mental conflict and affected my joy while being with them. When I honestly shared how I was struggling, my family was grateful to hear how I felt and immediately offered help. Because a good visit was important to me, I accepted this help. My daughter cooked a wonderful dinner for us that night while I engaged in my work. By allowing myself to let go of old ideas about how I should function as a mother while visiting my daughter, a new possibility arose. I empowered my daughter to help me, and we all experienced her delicious cooking. A generative conversation where I shared my struggle led to exploring solutions and created a new possibility for future visits. We now share cooking responsibilities when we get together.

While my personal example relates to juggling work and family life, we can apply the same skills to engage our family in supporting us when we are trying to lose weight or reach new health outcomes.

One of my patients, who wanted to combine the desire to exercise more and her love of spending time with her family, shared with them her desire to be more fit and proposed they buy new exercise equipment so they could enjoy improving their fitness as a family. The discussion that followed provided other family members the chance to contribute their ideas. They explored how the family could engage in various physical activities together and what equipment they might purchase. Rather than confining their ideas to what they could do inside the home, they brainstormed things such as biking and hiking vacations, options they had not considered before. The discussion benefited the whole family and enabled my patient to realize her desires.

Generative conversations, asking for what we need and want, and receiving the support we ask for are key components to our growth, well-being, and relationships. These capacities are powerful tools to help us overcome barriers as we strive to make changes in our life.

Dealing with Cultural Traditions & Older Family Members

We are all born into a particular cultural tradition and enter into a "molding process" that shapes us into culturally and socially acceptable beings. Our parents teach us to behave in ways that are socially acceptable so that we don't embarrass them in public or create havoc in private. They teach us skills to navigate the world with a sense of abundance or lack. Our parents want us to listen, remain safe, and learn their lessons. Acceptable behaviors are encouraged with praise or occasional treats, whereas bad behavior or inadequate performance are handled with timeouts, criticisms, or culturally acceptable physical punishment. Many of us may come from a patriarchal family system that socially conditions girls to be less assertive and to expect less possibilities than their male counterparts. Early conditioning establishes foundational structures, familial habits, and rituals that form our character, personality, our mindset, and expectations for our future. However, as children, we don't have the capacity to question or resist this molding process.

In order to flourish as adults, infants and children are hard-wired to expect touch, emotional connection, and a sense of belonging. As young children, we quickly learn how to maintain safety and acceptance from our clan. When we feel disapproval, we sense the potential for loss or disconnection from their support. If we don't receive what we need as children, it's devastating. We acquiesce or develop protective mechanisms and ways of being that may distance us from our needs and true authentic self. In general, though, we feel the positive affection of our elders and family, and we feel connected.

At some point, however, our family may reject or cut us off for making a decision that doesn't uphold the family or cultural values they taught us. This occurs in many families where an adult child comes out as gay or decides to switch gender identity. Or when an adult child marries someone outside the family's race or religion. Parents and extended family members may perceive such developments as dangerous or an expression of disloyalty. They may sense that if our choices lead us away from the family conditioning and become public news, they will be embarrassed, criticized, or rejected by their own social groups—members of their cultural, religious, and other communities that uphold the same norms and values. Just as they might be hurt by our choices, we are hurt by their reactions.

Bilateral silent agreements exist between parents and children so that the family, cultural, and ancestral norms survive. These expectations to believe and behave in particular ways are based on fear and survival. When we fulfill the expectations, we feel accepted, worthy of love, and a sense of belonging. When we feel like we don't belong because our unique characteristics are not valued, or we feel unworthy of love, our growth is actually stunted. This limits the potential for our extended family and us to consciously grow, appreciate variations among our family members, and experience unity.

Consider that our extended families or culture can be viewed as an external family system. This external family system is similar to our internal family system. Each member possesses particular mindsets, setpoints, assumptions and beliefs created by hard-wiring and prior experiences that protect family and cultural stability. In other words, our external family system is trying to protect its members, traditions, and us from danger, threats and change. When their emotional reactive system is ignited, they are triggered into fight-flight-freeze modes. They may react in such a way that we interpret their behavior as meanness to us or others. Even though such behaviors are unpleasant, we can manage these situations by implementing the same skills we learned to manage our internal family system when they are activated and triggered. We can choose to see our extended family members with compassion. And we can apply our developing generative conversation skills to deepen awareness and understanding of ideas and concerns different from our own. This may not be possible with certain family members or in some cultures. We may need to set appropriate boundaries to uphold our authentic values and find peace.

Case Study: Marion's Story

Marion, a patient, shared her experience of using generative conversation skills with her family about her self-identity change. A few years after she divorced a man who was abusive to her, she fell in love with a woman, and they decided to marry. In this relationship, Marion found joy and self-acceptance. She invested some time to prepare herself to talk with and inform her family of her upcoming marriage. Parts of her felt hesitant and afraid. She knew she was at risk of being rejected and exiled from them. She sensed that her decision to marry a woman would distress and embarrass her family. She calmed herself and extended compassion to those more fearful parts of herself, parts that craved her parents' approval.

When she met with her family, she vulnerably shared that she was gay and planned to marry her friend. She acknowledged the concern, sorrow, and humiliation her decision might cause for the family. She shared her recognition that it would be a process and take time for them to learn to see her differently. Despite this, Marion expressed her hope that their love for her and the love and connection she shared with them would be greater than the discomfort that might come from her decision. She asked for and emphasized how much their support would mean at this vulnerable time of making her private decision more public with the upcoming marriage. If they chose not to support her, she reminded them that they would miss her jokes, sense of humor, and silly holiday presents.

Marion was prepared, present, and grounded. She asked for what she wanted with heartful authenticity, appreciation for the others, and compassion for their situation. She avoided confrontation, transformed her fears, and garnered their attention and compassion. This kind of thoughtful and collaborative communication creates the likelihood of finding common ground, though it may take some time.

Ultimately, Marion's parents did not attend her wedding, but her siblings did. Even though Marion felt sad and hurt that her parents did not offer their support, she understood that their reactions were ancestral and reactive. She celebrated that she had the courage to have this generative conversation with her family and to authenticate this important and life-changing issue with honesty and integrity. She was able to discern and come to terms with what she could and could not change. Like Marion, we, as adults, can overcome obstacles that arise with our own external family system members. We can find our peace and wholeness when we live a life aligned with our truth and values and not that of others.

Always Remember:

Your worth is not negotiable.

You are enough just as you are.

You deserve to have wellness, health, love and abundance in your life.

What you eat, do, or choose, where you are from, and what others think about you does not affect your worth and value as a human in any way.

Trust that you are wise, mature, and able to nurture and care for yourself.

You choose and direct your path to wellness in all domains of your life.

The Influence of Our Social Network

Awareness is an essential step toward making and sustaining change. Our social network can impact our journey in positive or negative ways. It's important to evaluate the impact our social network has on us to make wise choices and create healthy boundaries. The more we increase our awareness, the better equipped we are to make decisions on how to prevent our social network from becoming an obstacle on our way to reaching our health goals.

When we make the decision to improve our health and lose weight, we may realize that some of our co-workers or neighbors are on a similar health journey. Since we are influenced by each other's weight, this awareness is beneficial to circumvent group influences that counteract our weight goals. Humans tend to gradually evolve their weight toward the weight of those around them. The group's weight becomes the new "normal," whether that weight is average, underweight, overweight, or obese. We also unconsciously seek friendships with people that look like us.

In addition, population data analysis shows that our weight tends to change towards that of our same-sex friends, our siblings, or our spouse/partner. Findings from a research study led by Dr. Nicholas Christakis published in the *New England Journal of Medicine* in 2007 demonstrate this. Among pairs of adult siblings, if one sibling became obese, the chance that the other would become obese increased by 40 percent. If one spouse became obese, the likelihood that the other spouse would also become obese increased by 37 percent. A person's chances of becoming obese increased by 57 percent if they had a friend who became obese. Pairs of friends and siblings of the same sex appeared to influence each other's weight gain more than pairs of the opposite sex. All in all, obesity has a social component and spreads among friends and family—the closer the connection, the greater the likelihood of this spread.

This study demonstrates how influential our social network can be on our behavior. If our social network has such an impact, then we can imagine the great benefit of obtaining *power partners*, individuals who have the same goals and drive, to support us and hold us accountable in reaching our weight loss and healthy living goals. Such partnerships can enable us to wisely overcome social pressures and ancestral tendencies. We can honor everyone in our social network but focus more on the power partners with similar aims to ours.

A powerful benefit of partnering with our intimate partners and family members to achieve our health goals is that couples and families tend to share a similar microbiome. The microbiome is affected by what we eat, so individuals living closely together in the same environment are likely to consume the same or similar food. It may be hard to lose weight if we are singly making changes because we share the same gut bacteria with our family. Stool samples reveal that couples and family members share the same microbiome bacteria. The interaction between diet and the wrong mix of gut bacteria can lead to obesity. When we change our diet, we change our microbiome. Involving the whole family in healthy living changes is helpful in order to make positive microbiome changes for everyone.

Dealing with Setbacks & Disappointments

Life is constantly changing around us. When the unexpected happens—a job loss, divorce, illness, or death—our security and safety may be challenged. Our ancestral response of fight-flight-freeze kicks in and disconnects us from ourselves. When triggered, the higher levels of thinking shut down, and we are less able to reflect and make conscious choices to effectively deal with the situation. How do we deal with the changes and challenges that occur? How do we set ourselves up for reacting less and responding more thoughtfully to difficulties and setbacks? How do we activate grit and hope?

Though counterintuitive to the reactive ancestral mind, ongoing daily self-care routines are crucial to handling the inevitable trials that come along. Healthy living routines, such as consistent meal schedules, exercise, and sleep habits are critical for our mind-body stability. We must care for our body systems and protect our personal circadian rhythm to nurture our being and lessen the burden of stress.

During difficult times, we can also connect with a supportive friend or power partner who will listen deeply and acknowledge our situation. A power partner or friend will reflect back to us a more accurate picture of who we are when stress overwhelms and confuses us. Such a friend boosts our confidence by reminding us of our grit and how we overcame challenges in the past. They will point out to us the new capacities, strengths, and resilience we've developed from previous trials. They will support us to shift our perspective from dwelling on the negative and recall joyful times to support us through the current challenges towards the future.

I have been the receiver of such support and also provided it to my family, friends, and patients. The capacities we have to lift each other up are powerful and life-giving. During these times, grace and spirit come together as hope. Hope is one of the greatest elements to restore equilibrium to our mind-body and activate our innate capacity to heal and overcome.

Developing the skills to train our minds to deal differently with setbacks and uncertainty is crucial to overcoming and growing from our experiences. A key component in how we manage setbacks and disappointments has to do with our perspective on the event. Many of us, particularly women, tend to blame ourselves when things are not working out as planned or things go wrong. We assume that something is our fault, that we are not enough, that we did not do enough or plan adequately, or don't know enough, or we don't meet our expectations. Research indicates women make more shame-based meanings of events than men. We automatically assume that we have a character flaw rather than seeing what happened as an opportunity for growth. self-derogatory thoughts, self-criticism, and guilt lead to a sense of despair and helplessness. It's important to avoid staying in negative spaces which help no one.

Rather than blaming and reprimanding ourselves when things don't go our way, we can practice curiosity. Through curiosity we can ask questions that help us evaluate the circumstances that led to the problem. We can identify potential opportunities for different approaches and actions that can be employed in the future. We can learn to avoid this unnecessary type of disempowerment and instead use self-agency over what we can actually control and validate our efforts. Despite our best intentions, we do not control outcomes.

You don't know what you don't know. So, another skill is to recognize when you don't know something and be able to seek out resources to solve a problem or accomplish a particular task. We can wonder, "how can we acquire the information and get the support we need?" There is no shame in honestly admitting, "I cannot do this *yet* because I have not learned how to do it." This is different than saying to yourself, "I cannot do this because I'm stupid and incapable." We cannot be expected to know how to solve problems or perform tasks when we have not received the training or had sufficient experience. We can practice reminding ourselves that mistakes are opportunities for growth, learning new skills, and training the brain to respond calmly. What we say to ourselves matters and creates positive or negative outcomes. Curiosity is a powerful virtue that brings new awareness and empowers us to face our challenges in a more expansive manner and explore new possibilities to deal with challenges and difficulties.

Boundaries: What's Okay, What's Not Okay

While it is possible to evolve personal relationships to where they are not causing harm, occasionally, there are circumstances in which, despite our best effort, an individual or a group continue to erode our wellness. How do we protect ourselves from individuals, activities and environments that compromise our health and well-being?

Most of us would agree certain behaviors are never acceptable. Physical, sexual, and emotional threats and abuse are wrong. No one wants to be hurt, debased, disenfranchised, unwelcomed, relentlessly criticized, or ignored by another. Unfortunately, these behaviors happen most often between family members. One in three women and one in four men will experience physical, emotional, or sexual violence by a family member. My patients who experience these painful circumstances are often afraid to share with others what is happening in their own homes. They feel ashamed, helpless, and stuck in circumstances that are depleting them, and they don't know where to turn or how to reach out. They need help from family, friends or authorities to overcome fear and access their innate courage to act on their behalf for their own wellness. They must avoid or move away from their abuser. Period.

But domestic violence is a very complicated and sensitive issue. What may seem sensible to do does not always occur. The possibility of setting boundaries is often not considered when the ancestral brain is chronically and constantly activated by fear and self-preservation mode.

Those of us who have learned and have more practice setting boundaries are fortunate. We have the privilege of learning and setting boundaries as a way of expressing what is okay and what is not okay in our relationships, work environments, and communities. We can continue to learn how to establish boundaries with individuals who have deeply hurt us. The ability to create physical distance is a vital step to our empowerment.

However, even with our boundaries in place, we may continue to feel victimized or damaged. Perhaps we are holding onto grudges and resentments against the person who caused us harm. We may feel 'less than' or unworthy, isolated, and ashamed. According to neuroscientist and pharmacologist, Candace Pert, Ph.D., negative emotions can release chemicals that damage our body and its essential systems. When an emotion is triggered, it causes a neuroelectric signal that moves throughout the body.

How do we consciously free ourselves from this inner emotional turmoil? I believe we can have more light and abundance by striving to have compassion for ourselves which opens our hearts and gives access to our spirit wisdom. Having more positive regard and compassion for ourselves is the antidote.

Meditation, as explored earlier, is one of the tools we have to release inner grievances. Many may struggle with forgiving unjust and harmful behaviors. However, when we forgive ourselves or those who have harmed us, we are not forgetting what happened or accepting harmful actions. Rather, forgiveness is about giving ourselves the gift of releasing the burden and grip of an unfortunate occurrence in the past. When we witness our feelings and acknowledge our suffering with compassion, especially in front of a mature presence—a therapist, power partner, or our own wise and centered adult self, we can experience profound transformation and freedom. When we move from shame to self-acceptance and from victim to self-empowerment, we have the moral authority and wisdom to help others in similar situations.

Sometimes we may behave in ways that are not consistent with our current identity, vision, or higher values. When this happens, become curious and ask, what is happening here? How old is this part of me that is acting out? What do they really need? What motivates them to do this? Analyze the behavior and explore solutions. For example, one of my patients, a successful business owner who is trying to lose weight, shared that she stops at Carvel's ice cream shop when no one is in the car with her. She finds it thrilling to get away with doing this but then feels that she can't be trusted. Another patient describes eating a whole bag of cookies and then feeling guilty afterwards. Both of these behaviors are child-like or primitive rebellious or soothing reactions of disenfranchised younger parts of ourselves who felt controlled, criticized, shamed or untrusted. Emotional states, certain events, or stress triggers can bring out these younger hurt or isolated inner family members. Binge-eating and other disordered eating behaviors, are evidence that a part of us is in great need for self-nurturing and self-love. Recognizing this self-suffering, why they exist, and their mode of operating gives entry to self-compassion and a path to healing. Knowing this can help us, without shame, get the help we need from an experienced therapist and others that have overcome this.

Similarly, some may have trouble managing alcohol, unable to stop after the first drink, or end up with a DUI, or hospitalized for overindulgence. Alcohol abuse or addictions have a genetic and biologic drive for them. However, the onset of these can also be traced to younger parts of us that felt isolated. They lacked nurturing, love, sense of belonging or approval, and found that alcohol soothed them or checked them out from their suffering. Regardless of the origins of the problem, alcohol abuse and addiction are a signal that it is time to set stronger boundaries with ourselves. This is one of the times that it is essential to establish zero tolerance to exposing ourselves to certain foods, drinks or objects that trigger us into losing control. Again, curiosity and compassion for ourselves or another helps to counteract the guilt that may trigger another episode of straying from upholding our values and desire to feel whole or well.

We are social creatures influenced by the habits and behaviors of our friends. Being aware of how our friends, not just family members, may trigger our insecurities is integral in our process of making changes in ourselves. This can be particularly challenging when striving to make changes, transform, and become grounded in a new healthy identity. When we spend time with a friend, sometimes old patterns can be triggered, such as unconsciously seeking the approval of others. Say a friend suggests splitting a dessert while out for dinner, even when they know we are striving to maintain a healthy diet. This puts us in a precarious situation because we don't want to *disappoint them.* In another example, we may find that a friend or co-worker triggers an old pattern of feeling like we are never enough as we are. They may judge our particular journey to healthier living and point out what's wrong with what we are doing, so *we feel discouraged.* We need to limit the time we spend with people who trigger our insecurities and instead cultivate social relationships with people who bring out the best in us and encourage us to live according to the changes we are seeking until we are firmly established and grounded in our new identity.

Creating boundaries is a vital skill to cultivate and use without feeling doubtful or ashamed for doing so. We establish boundaries to protect our children. We use outlet covers so they don't electrocute themselves. We teach them to stay away from the street and only cross after looking both ways. We feed them and put them to bed on time. We keep our children away from bullies and abusive people. We can and must extend this same kind of protection to nurture ourselves. If we have trouble doing so, we can seek the aid of trained professionals who can help us evolve and overcome habits and behaviors that take away our joy and wholeness.

Learning how to identify what boundaries we need and then carrying through and establishing those boundaries can help us to achieve our health goals in an unstoppable way. This skill set enables us to live more fully and joyfully. Some additional examples that demonstrate we are becoming more competent at establishing healthy boundaries include the following:

- Establishing and committing to self-care time.
- Learning to delegate tasks, chores, and other responsibilities.
- Asking for help and resources.
- Saying "no" to requests that interfere with the time you have scheduled for self-care or if the task or event is not aligned with your current values and goals.
- Recognizing that we have control of our actions and our attitudes, independent of what others do or say.
- Becoming curious about what the circumstances were when something does not go our way or when we see ourselves acting in ways that no longer represent what we value or who we truly are.

When we schedule and strive to honor regular appointments with ourselves for self-care, we need to say "no" to what might come along to disrupt that appointment. We are saying "no" in order to say "yes" to caring for our well-being. Appointments and commitments with ourselves must become non-negotiable. We must realize these appointments are as important, if not more so, than any other appointment. We must see these self-care appointments as if we are meeting a very special person who will save our life. We, in fact, are. *We are that important.*

We have the capacity to learn multiple skills to overcome obstacles to our growth and transformation. Key skills are *curiosity* and *compassion,* which are essential tools to deploy in all aspects of healing and creating *boundaries* to support ourselves, achieve our health goals, and maintain our healthy values.

My Loving-Kindness Wish for You

May you feel calm and centered
May you have conversations that heal
May you feel your worth and know you belong
May you feel heard, seen, valued, trusted
May you nurture yourself
and let yourself be held
by your essence and love.

Meditation to Enhance Your Journaling

Please scan the QR Code with your Smartphone
or follow this link: https://youtu.be/SuLBWdAHyq8

Journaling for Transformation

We are all human. We are all imperfect. We are all in this process together. We are all asking different questions as to where we are going and how to do it better. We all come from the same earth, are made of the same substance, and are subject to our shared ancestral core.

After reading this chapter, can you identify all the skills discussed to overcome obstacles to growth? Which skills can you use right away to make your life better?

- Can you explain to someone what a generative conversation is?
- Can you think of opportunities to use these conversations to support yourself and others to be well?
- What obstacles affect or may affect your capacity to maintain momentum to support your wellness?
- Is your home environment supportive of your vision? How can you make it more supportive?
- Is your work environment supporting your goals? What changes need to be made?
- Are your relationships nurturing and supportive of your growth?
- How do you handle setbacks or disappointments? Can you identify a way you can manage them better?
- What creative ways can you come up with to protect yourself and your growth?
- If you cannot change what is occurring in your life, can you be with what is? Can you find a way to validate and nurture yourself with more compassion? How so?
- Can you create new activities to engage in with friends that do not involve eating pizza or pastries? Have you considered hiking, roller skating, going to the movies or bowling?
- How will others benefit from your becoming more vibrant and healthier?
- What changes are you empowered to make in your life after reading this chapter?

Chapter 9

Spirituality for a Healthy Lifespan & Soul-Satisfying Life

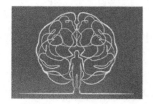

The keystone to health and wellness comes from allowing Spirit and Soul to imbue us with health and life.

While theologians and philosophers invest years of study to explore the existence of the spirit and soul, we all possess the power of imagination and creativity to explore these realities. Though difficult concepts to comprehend, higher levels of thought, and often surrender, allow us to behold spirit-energy and the soul, that which is beyond our vision, that which calls and directs us to our highest expression of being.

In this final chapter, I want to share my personal views and understandings of the importance of spirit and the soul to our well-being, not as a theologian or member of a religious community, but as a human being, a physician, and a mind-body expert. I recognize that my opinions may at times be more biologic—and less religion-based, but this is how I have logically come to embrace the transcendent and powerful presence of soul and spirit in my life.

Spirit, Spirit-Energy & Spirituality

I view **Spirit** as the nonphysical and energetic part of our being that animates and gives life and breath to our body. All beings carry this essential energetic ingredient. This energy is invisible yet quantifiable, consistent with the first law of thermodynamics in physics that states, energy is neither created nor destroyed. Spirit simply is. I think of spirit as that single point of energy from the Big Bang—a single point of energy from nowhere that exploded and expanded into the expanse of the universe we have today, and is energetically carried through our genetic material or DNA.

The Big Bang energy is carried by each one of us. We start as a single cell containing the DNA of our parents and generations before them. This energy that came through our parent's union remains with us throughout life. I call the energy from Spirit, **spirit-energy** and view it as the source of our vitality. Others may refer to this as the life force.

This spirit-energy gives animation and vibrancy to our being. Though, as we age, the capacity to express this energetic vibrancy declines as we physically age and the body experiences diseases of aging. Diseases of the brain or nervous system, like Alzheimer's, ALS, and MS, damage the brain and nervous system. My mother had Alzheimer's disease, and her damaged brain prevented her physically from showing the presence of her spirit and spirit-energy. Nonetheless, I know with deep awareness that my mother's spirit was fully there until her death. Similarly, after heart attacks and lung damage, the body's capacity to use oxygen so that mitochondria can make energy is limited, making it hard to move or do anything that requires effort without extreme fatigue or shortness of breath. The point here is that lacking physical energy, or not being able to express it, does not equate to an absence of spirit or loss of spirit-energy. Spirit and spirit-energy, regardless of how it is expressed throughout our lives, only departs at the time we physically die. I honor being alive and the presence of spirit.

Throughout our lives, we have the capacity to access this spirit-energy when we are centered, and our mind-body unit is aligned. When we are connected to our spirit-energy, we can rest and recharge our mind-body's operating systems. I have been able to personally access this energy and be in this awareness during meditation or while communing with nature. When we commune with others we are energetically interacting with each other's spirit-energies. Don't you feel energized when you have spent time with a dear friend who sees you, makes you laugh, and feel glad you are alive? Connecting to other energy fields, like nature, is life-giving for me, and reconnects me to my origin and own healing energy. I feel a sense of aliveness, keen awareness, creativity and hope. I'm connected to my own power, resilience and grit.

Nature, great personal interactions, and meditation are ways that I connect to spirit-energy. I have also found that professional energy work is very valuable. Energy healing has been used for thousands of years in multiple cultures. Since childhood, I have reconnected to my own energy and healing capacities through various energy workers. As an adult, polarity, craniosacral, myofascial, acupuncture practitioners have tangibly helped me restore or reconnect to my energy system and remove blocks to the flow of energy through the body, mind and spirit.

While spirit-energy can be easily accessed when we are calm, our own emotions and day-to-day stressful existence can disconnect us from ourselves and Spirit. As a result, we feel less energized. Stress, negative interactions, and the feelings triggered have us reacting to the day-to-day details and put us on guard. When we are continuously in our heads with worry, distraction, stress, and fear, our mind-body functions separate to go into flight-fight-freeze survival mode. When we are in this stress state, we are more reactive. In this space, it's difficult to find the patience or the right response or solution that the situation calls for. When we are in the headspace of flight fight survival mode, we cannot connect with higher consciousness or to the power of our spirit's wisdom, this is because the mind and body are not aligned. Mind-body alignment and re-connection is required to access higher consciousness and spirit. These are exactly the times when it matters most to take a timeout, just a few minutes to sit and breathe, physically feeling our body breathing and sitting in our energetic space. When we take a mindful timeout, we reconnect our mind to the physicality of our body. This realignment allows us to reconnect to the power of our spirit and life force.

Some refer to the concept of Spirit and spirit-energy as God, Goddess, or the Universe. Different religions and people throughout the world ascribe a particular name to this energy. Regardless of the words we use to describe it, Spirit is a universal concept shared and experienced to varying degrees by most of humanity.

Spirituality is the capacity to explore the transcendent and sacred. It is the ability to question and experience that which connects us to life, ourselves, others, nature, and this moment. Spirituality allows us to belong and be part of something greater than ourselves, to concern ourselves with the spirit or soul, to possess a consciousness that recognizes or senses something beyond our material existence. Spirituality involves exploring the meaning or purpose of life without necessarily aligning ourselves with a particular religion, though belonging to a religion is a source of spiritual connection. Spirituality can be life-saving, as it can make us feel that we belong to a larger consciousness and universal humanity even when we are physically alone. Spirituality allows for a connection to spirit-energy and to our soul. This is the place where we find the hope, courage, and resilience to overcome our darkest times. This concept may or may not be related to religiosity.

Many patients in my office are spiritual, but are not connected to a religious practice or group. Spirituality is extremely important to humans, particularly when we are experiencing threatening illnesses or are facing end-of-life issues and personal loss. Belonging to a religious faith, as a source of spiritual connection, has been shown to improve our mental health and helps young people feel a sense of belonging and a part of a group during the tempestuous times of the teenage years.

Conventional medicine has focused on the body and mind health, not on spiritual health. It is now trying to reconcile itself with and revise its view of how to incorporate spirituality into medicine to help patients cope with the health challenges they face. Spiritual health matters because people view illnesses and make meaning of them using spiritual beliefs and perspectives of our socialized mind. If spiritual health is not considered, we fail to understand how much of our lack of wellness (with and without disease), burnout, job dissatisfaction, loneliness, sarcasm, and annihilation, are all distresses or ailments of the spirit and soul.

Giving ourselves the gift to be spiritual, to be curious, to develop a spiritual practice that seeks to honor what we need, what gives us meaning, and what we value in life, is one of the most powerful actionable gifts we can give ourselves in this lifetime. It is empowering and freeing. Wouldn't it be nice to be free and feel that we are well, that we belong, and that we are empowered to make decisions based on this that heals us? What are your thoughts on all this?

The Soul

Spirituality allows for the possibility that the **soul** exists. Many people consider that the soul moves on when we die. Some people pray for their own and others souls. We also ascribe emotional depth and wisdom to the concept of soul, and might describe someone as soulful. When I was younger, I considered the soul as the keeper of our goodness or our badness, the part of us that experiences the consequences of our earthly life. I believed that when people died, souls hung out at the cemetery, went to heaven or to hell, or were recycled and reborn carrying residue from a prior life. I always felt empathy for the soul since it, and not us, ultimately paid the price of our existence.

Over the years, the soul has been a topic of great personal curiosity, contemplation, and growth for me. I want to tell you my understanding of the soul by sharing personal stories that led me to embrace its presence in my life, and to focus on using its qualities to create a more enriched life. I am convinced that the soul is a life-giving source of health and wellness. The soul is that place of light and wisdom within us that is deeply attached to our life experience and connects us to spirit. The soul is a conduit between our physical and outer experience and inner spirit-energy. The soul is that place of reconciliation and wholeness within us humans. The soul is the keeper of our personal journey and mythology. I believe that a lot of ailments that we don't have an answer for are distresses of the soul or disconnection from it.

The Soul as Our House of Reflection

The first time I encountered a more nuanced idea of the soul occurred when I was an intern. For 27 days, during my first year of working as a doctor after medical school, I took care of a patient who had lupus. At times I felt she was better; at times I felt she was worse. At the end, when all of her systems were failing, we became emotionally close during this intimate time. Toward the end of her journey, I had to tell her that we had exhausted her medical treatment options. "I'm still going to try my best, you know, to be here for you," I said. I held her hands and she held mine back with such gratitude. That afternoon, I left her room for a short time and when I came back, she was gone.

Her death devastated me. Here I was, at the start of my career, suddenly realizing that helping people die was part of my job and questioning my capacity to do so. How could I believe that I was so ready to serve as a doctor yet so unprepared to deal with death? I became deeply sad, actually depressed. I started to believe I didn't have what it takes to be a good doctor. At that point, I was young and didn't understand the complexities of grief after death or how to process this grief to move on and grow from experiencing loss.

Thankfully, Dr. Michael Karpf, chief of my internal medicine residency team, encouraged me to begin psychotherapy, which I found incredibly helpful. I also read and contemplated *The Care of the Soul* by Thomas Moore, a book that transformed my life. I learned that depression, the very dark space I found myself in, was actually a cry from my soul inviting me to enter its house of reflection. In this contemplative space I could sit and be with my emotions and grief, clarifying and making meaning of what had occurred. That's when I understood that depression can be a distress call from our soul, an opportunity to tend to ailments that challenge who we are and our existence so we can build resilience for the future. Depression can be a healing pathway for us, and our soul has a way to reach us, to challenge us and inspire reflection, allowing for the making of meaning and for negative experiences to be sublimated to growth.

These early experiences deepened my interest in the interrelationship between mental health and physical wellness in relation to our spirit and soul. As the years went by, I better understood and accepted that suffering and loss are a common part of the human condition. The grief we feel humbles us, unites us, and adds depth to our lives. From the understanding of our shared humanity, our compassion and understanding of one another increases.

Full circle and years later, I was part of a Yale University medical faculty team that taught Dr. Rachel Naomi Remen's "Healer's Art" course to medical students. Rachel N. Remen, a pediatrician, gained global attention as a best-selling author and teacher of integrative medicine. Her book *Kitchen Table Wisdom*, a soulful depiction of healing in doctor and patient interactions, has been translated into 21 languages. The "Healer's Art" course is now included in medical student curriculum in medical schools throughout the United States. The course teaches the importance of self-care, how to deal heartfully with death and grief, and to recognize the dignity of our work as doctors in the service and care of patients. I have become an expert at teaching what I wish I had known that first month of my internal medicine internship.

The Soul as a Companion & Resource

Years ago, I had to have a lumbar fusion. I had been a gymnast earlier in my life and unknowingly injured my spine. Soon after I got home from the surgery, I could not stand up. Every time I stood up, my feet and legs felt as if they were burning in a live fire. I dealt with this experience for days hoping it would go away. It did not. Pain became an ever-present and unwanted companion. I was convinced that something had gone wrong with the surgery. Typical pain medications knocked me out but were ineffective at decreasing the type of nerve pain that I was having.

I was readmitted to the hospital. After an emergency CT scan, the radiologist informed me that all of the rods, pedicles and screws were exactly where they should be. There was nothing wrong. Though the operation was a success, I, the patient, felt as if I were dying at the stake. How could this be? How could there be nothing visibly wrong, when I was suffering so much pain?

That night, in the twilight, I imagined myself living without energy and in pain for the rest of my life. Devastated, I held on to the hospital bed railing as I wavered between disbelief and drowsiness. At some point, I accepted this new reality and surrendered. Just then, though no one was in my room, a serious yet neutral voice awakened me. "You need steroids," I heard. I pinched my arm. I was not hallucinating. "You need steroids," I heard once again. This firm voice could not be dismissed.

The next morning, Dr. Hilary Onyiuke, the neurosurgeon and a colleague of mine, confirmed the findings of the CT scan showing that everything was in the right place and said that I could go home. "I believe I need steroids," I respectfully stated. He and his team explained that they never prescribe steroids after lumbar fusions because steroids can interfere with the fusion. I remained firm and requested a prescription. They agreed as long as I signed a waiver accepting the risk of non-fusion and absolving them of any responsibility for the therapy that was not standard of care. I signed the waiver.

For the first time in a week, after receiving an intravenous dose of dexamethasone, I was able to stand up. I cried with joy as I walked to the window. I saw the red and yellow colors of the fall trees. I felt such joy to see those colors and walked out of the hospital that day full of hope, filled with gratitude for my soul's wisdom.

Even though I was a doctor, a hormone doctor no less, I was amazed at and thankful for the power of steroids. The treatment, brief in duration, quieted the unusual degree of inflammation that squeezed my nerve roots each time I stood up. This pressure on the nerve roots caused the burning sensation. The use of steroids relieved the pressure without interfering with the ultimate outcome of the surgery, and the bone fusion occurred. Nowadays, more than a decade later, patients routinely receive a dose of steroids, like dexamethasone, when undergoing orthopedic procedures.

This remains one of the most awe-filled spiritual experiences in my life. I believe that the soul is uniquely related to us and our individual experiences. My soul had access to medical knowledge that my doctors and I did not have. Something within me and beyond my consciousness had a knowingness and intuition that led to this intentional and powerful healing experience. I was awed and filled with hope which re-connected me to my spirit-energy. When I tell this story to our medical students, they, and a little part of me, still ask, "Who spoke?"

The Soul is the Keeper of Our Mythology

I've come to believe that the soul is the home of our personal journey and the keeper of our mythology, joys, and sorrows. The soul is the connection between what happens in our outside world, in our mind-body unit, and the spirit-essence always present within us. To this day I address both the mind and body together in my medical practice to help patients cultivate hope and uncover the spiritual meaning of illness in their lives. I learned this by reading Thomas Moore's book, *Care of the Soul*, whose insights made a powerful impression on me and informed the way that I practice medicine. Moore emphasizes that our personal story, our mythology, plays a great role in how we interact and relate with others. The creation of this myth emerges from our family, our religion, and the various institutions that shape us and socialize our mind. Our culture, beliefs, education, sufferings and successes shape our mythology, which in turn, influences our capacity to heal and our understanding of what an illness can mean for us. Though we are visibly functioning at the mind-body level, our myth and the meaning we make about who we are, has great power over the outcome of our health, wellness, and other domains in life.

I have learned that I can't help my patients if I don't connect with them. If I don't understand their personal story or the meaning that the illness has for them, prescribing the correct medicine will not be enough to meet them where they need to be met. If I connect at a deeper level, at a soul level, I can then sense and understand the greater context of what the illness means to them and how involved they will be in their healing process. When this happens, I can truly help.

Nurturing the Soul: Finding Dignity & Meaning in Our Work

In recent years, excessive red tape and documentation have hurt patient-doctor interactions. Doctors have less and less time to meet patients where they need to be met, or to establish these types of healing connections. For us doctors, our work as physicians has been about human connection and serving others, but it's hard to serve others when we lose agency over how we do our work and interact with our patients. In addition, doctors and support staff waste valuable hours trying to get approval from medical insurance companies for medicines that patients need. These companies, who seek profit, often deny, make it difficult, or don't cover needed medications. This creates deep dissatisfaction for patients who do not feel served and for doctors who cannot serve well, despite hours of work that also keeps them from their families and what they value. We become depleted. This reality leads us to question the meaning, purpose, and even the dignity of our work as physicians. More than ever doctors are experiencing burnout, disconnection and disempowerment, depression, and sadly suicide. The first four are ailments of the soul and the latter the consequences of not being able to tend it.

I believe this is a crisis moment for our current medical system. This is why I, as an integrative physician, feel so strongly that a holistic human-centered approach is needed to create the future medical system. Hopefully this will be a place where goals to heal are aligned by using a human-centered approach that empowers patients to feel heard and served, and doctors to have self-agency and dignity in their work.

My own internship and resident years were very difficult. The focus was on saving lives through caring for the sick and learning the skills to diagnose and treat various conditions with medicines or surgery. Other residents and I sometimes wondered how we could maintain the inspiration that led us to serve as doctors. We felt challenged to maintain empathy and compassion when we had to detach to complete our work with objectivity. Reminding ourselves that we were providing valuable services to support others gave meaning to our work as young physicians and enabled us to embrace the value and dignity of our work. I began to see that I was engaged in a process of nurturing and developing my soul and expanding my own mythology through my work as a doctor, especially when I faced challenges later in life.

Jobs, in and outside the field of medicine, are complex places, whether we work with people or machines. At times, our work environments and tasks are challenging, potentially risky, and even hazardous. We may work in toxic environments that stress our bodies, our minds, and/or our emotions. We all need to feel that our presence and work matter, that we belong and contribute. Sometimes we are not seen, heard, or valued so stop seeing the purpose of our work. Many of us don't recognize the importance, at these times, of connecting to our values and personal needs, talking to those we love. This is when we need to give ourselves time to regroup and reflect in order to give language to how we feel, so we can take steps to change our situation.

How can we proactively face these dissatisfying conditions in an empowering way? How can we cultivate qualities and care for our own souls to bring forward the dignity needed to engage in work productively? What do we have to do to find meaning in our work? How can we contribute to improve the environment we work and live in?

A few powerful solutions are to befriend and care for ourselves, create clear and intentional boundaries between work and our private life, and acknowledge the soulful need to have a job that gives us dignity. When we cannot change our job or its culture easily, imagine adopting the mindset that work is a sacred task that we can engage in with self-respect, presence, and the intention to serve. A mindset such as this can satisfy and renew us. A mindset such as this can enable us to engage productively in work as a way to care for our own souls. Maya Angelou said, "If your work is not satisfying, you are not meeting your soul's need."

The soul is the place where unimaginable energetic potential exists and calls us to be and connect to our highest and best selves. This is our house of reflection. We can reflect and reconnect to that which we value and gives meaning to our lives. We can assess our capacities, skills and values and seek out work that aligns with our gifts and talents, work that is life-giving and meaningful. There, we can reconnect to our wholeness and return to what inspires us to become our highest selves.

Additionally, we can consult and collaborate with others to support us in making these determinations rather than struggle alone. It may mean we have to have the courage to leave work that does not give us life or dignity, especially when we no longer can show up and give our best to fulfill our highest calling to serve others. One way I chose to do this was to eliminate medical insurance payments and their limitations from my work as a doctor. This was a difficult decision but it empowered me to spend more time and connect with patients and serve their needs. This also gave me the time I need to use my skills to the highest level. My patients now feel that they get value and results from our interaction, and I feel that I've reclaimed my agency, my dignity, my well-being. I took a stance to nurture what I value and my soul with my work.

Relationships, Longevity & Soulfulness

Our soulful connections remain alive and are part of the essence of who we are.

The soul grows and is nurtured by our interactions with the people around us and the environment. My grandmother, Celita, was the adult who most nurtured and unconditionally loved me while I was growing up in Cuba. The experiences I shared with her, early and later in my life, bring warmth to my heart and a smile to my face even now. She would take me on horse-drawn coach rides and we would have wonderful talks. She asked me a lot of questions about how I felt about things or viewed them. She treated me as if I were a most interesting and important person. She made me feel I mattered to her. She took me to operas and my first film in Cuba, *Pinocchio*. She let me be and eat when I wanted. Her meals were so healthy, fresh, and delicious. I felt so welcomed and happy to be in her home. Now, as an adult, I take coach rides whenever I can. I always cook and create space to make people feel that they belong. I am so deeply grateful that she was and continues to be in my memories and personal expressions in my life. I think she gave soulfulness to my life. If the soul lives on, this is a way in which it does so. We remember the people that filled our lives with joy and gave us a sense that we belonged and mattered to them.

My grandmother Celita passed when she was 101 years old, a centenarian. A small percentage of the billions of people live to 100 and beyond. What does it take to live into our nineties and beyond? What are the secrets? Individuals and researchers throughout the world are engaged in these questions. As a doctor, I am interested in and committed to uncovering and sharing the secrets of longevity. We can learn from my grandmother and reflect on the Blue Zone areas of the world, areas of the world where the average lifespan of people living there appears to be longer than the rest of the world.

Researchers study the Blue Zone areas of the world because of the longevity of their inhabitants. Blue Zone areas are located in Ikaria, Greece; Loma Linda, California; Sardinia, Italy; Okinawa, Japan and Nicoya, Costa Rica. The common thread people share in Blue Zones is a healthy diet (mostly plant-based), active lifestyles, and multigenerational, interconnected families. These communities display the qualities that nurture soul-filled lives. Everyone feels a sense of purpose and belonging. Elders are admired and consulted for their wisdom. Relationships at every age are valued and support individuals to have satisfying lives.

Relationships with those near and far can increase our joy. We can treasure the memories of relatives and friends long after they are gone. We can visualize special people from our past and those who live at a distance to uplift our spirits. I treasure the memories I hold close of my grandmother Celita. These memories uplift my soul. They provide substance, purpose, and meaning to my life. They are a vital part of my own soulfulness.

Soulfulness enhances our relationships with ourselves, others, and the universe. Likewise, pondering our relationships with ourselves, others, and the universe proactively and spiritually can expand our soulfulness...and according to Blue Zones research, perhaps our longevity.

Developing the Qualities of the Soul

The soul, for me, embodies the idea of the great mother who unconditionally loves and accepts us. The soul, like the great mother, embraces our light and our shadow sides with equanimity. All our qualities and imperfections, our goodness and our shadow coexist as parts of our wholeness. The soul knows that we are not perfect, ever. Good and bad are inevitable and exist in each of us. The journey to become whole is the work of our soul. The soul invites us to reach our highest potential as humans and to embrace our wholeness. We begin to understand the inevitability of the *good* and the *bad* inside us, the messiness and complexities and the paradoxes.

In our journey to understand what soulfulness might mean, we can take the time to look for qualities of the soul in ourselves and others. Noting the development of qualities like acceptance, compassion and dignity as we realize our own and one another's imperfections and complexities. We can acknowledge the quality of patience as the soul continues to serve as the keeper of our hurts, losses, and sadness. We can also identify and develop numerous other qualities, like presence, compassion, acceptance, integrity, wisdom, abundance, knowingness, unboundedness, reflection, connection, courage, equanimity, and gratitude.

We have incredible capacity to exercise generosity and compassion as we journey towards accepting our complexities within this space of wholeness. When we embrace our wholeness, we come from a place of abundance. We stop ourselves from the tendency to compare ourselves with one another. We realize that we are not lacking. Rather, we see ourselves as enough and having enough. We see and reflect back the goodness in others. We give from our soulful heart, even if we perceive we don't have very much to offer. We receive help, affection, and love from others.

As discussed earlier, meditation and the deeper alignment of our mind-body-spirit can help us work with disenfranchised parts of ourselves, the parts we perceive as darker and more problematic. We can accept these parts, acknowledge their existence, their suffering and efforts to hide us from shame. We can accept the disenfranchised parts and integrate them into our wholeness. This kind of self-compassion is an act of the soul that heals us.

The Role of the Soul During Dark Times

The soul's capacity to remember all that we have endured makes it the holder of our suffering. The soul holds all of our heart's journeys, including the trials and calamities. So often trials and tragedies enable us to evolve and grow, just like the lotus flower grows from the dirt and mud. However, we don't always realize the growth ahead while enduring the pain of the suffering. This was the case for one of my patients who confided that she had closed her heart a long time ago when she lost a relationship with a beloved partner. She made the decision to stop listening to music. Music was a direct path and opened the door to her soul. She didn't want to revisit the space that held her suffering until she was ready.

So often as we deal with and strive to face life's trials, we also struggle with depression, a dark tunnel. We may find it difficult, maybe even impossible, to believe that there is a light at the end of that tunnel. While in this dark tunnel, we tend to remember and reflect on all the times that we failed, times that we were humiliated, times when we didn't think that we could stand up and times when we lost someone, and we kept on losing them, every day, for years.

Depression causes or is caused by our inability to cope with a major or perceived stressor and by mal-alignment of the mind-body unit. This mal-alignment creates chemical imbalances and disconnection from our source, our spirit-energy. When we are sad or depressed, we have less energy, motivation or desire. During these times we need the help of others to remind us of the qualities we possess, our goodness, and what we mean to them. We need to know that we belong. Receiving this kind of generative feedback helps us to reconnect with our soul.

When I was very young, the Cuban government seized everything our family owned because my father refused to further communist teachings at the medical school. The government ordered that the University of Havana fire my father from his job as a professor of Pediatrics at the University and sent us to live in Oriente, the most eastern Cuban province. Then the government assigned my father a job hours away from our family, separating us. During one of my summer visits to him, my father offered me illuminating guidance. He shared that while people can take everything from you in the physical world, they cannot take your knowledge, your higher thoughts, your hopes, or your attitude. These are always in our domain. These qualities of character, he told me, are what ultimately define us. We need to hold on to these inner qualities and values to survive. Later, when I looked back on this conversation, I realized that my father provided the advice that we would need to survive and succeed in another country.

Though it took us a decade to leave Cuba after Castro arrived, my father's guidance contributed to my becoming a successful immigrant and survivor. I often reflect on how deeply I listened to my father. Though I was young and unable to help my disenfranchised father, the fact that I was a listening presence gave us both the spirit-energy we needed to endure. The qualities and values of the soul my father had emphasized provided the courage and grit to move through the difficulties in our new life in America. At the time, we may not have realized that our conversation back in Cuba would contribute to my carrying our story and message forward to the next generation.

Such meaningful and soulful interactions create a family's mythology, hope for the future, and the stories and lasting life experiences that are shared through the generations. These spiritually enlightened and energizing interactions teach us how to take care of ourselves, cultivate resilience and courageously take the next step forward. We access the fortitude to wake up and show up every day, even when we feel emotionally naked, vulnerable and disconnected. These connections enable us to slowly find our way. We begin to sense our existence matters. We reconnect our hurting and healing mind-body unit to spirit-energy through our souls and soulful interactions with those we love, especially in the midst of challenges. The soul remembers and knows how to bring us back to our wholeness, ourselves and our shared lives.

What Happens to the Soul?

We are all so familiar with these questions. What is the soul? How do our experiences influence the soul? What happens to the soul after death? Questions about the nature and mystery of the soul are intriguing. We may have ideas and thoughts at one time in our life that evolve over time. Some of us may have little time or interest in pondering such questions, but often the loss of a loved one will cause us to reflect.

I believe that the soul grows and is nurtured by our experiences. Sometimes I believe that when we are young, we are less soulful than when we are older and might be very soulful. However, we have all met young people who appear to have old and wise souls. Tragically, some people may never become soulful because they were not or could not be nurtured to develop spiritual qualities or simply have more interest in their physical lives.

Energy is neither created nor destroyed. That is true of our spirit-energy as well, in my mind. Is this true of the soul? Does the soul end with death? I have sometimes considered that the soul, being so related to our physical reality, may die and end when we do. Other times, as I was taught early on, I have thought the parts of the soul upon death connect to the souls that have left before us. For example, I sense my grandmother's love and soulfulness in me, I truly feel her energy within me. Still, at other times I believe that when we physically die, the soul may go to other places like heaven, or may be reincarnated in other spaces, or may stay around to help those it knew in this life. I think my mother stayed a long time to do this. Other bodhisattvas have done the same.

Who knows what truly happens to the soul upon death? I don't, but I remain curious and hope I will continue to reflect and develop more knowledge about the mystery and nature of the soul as I age.

Grace

Grace is the highest expression of the union of spirit-energy with the soul. The Universal spirit-energy is given to us at birth and unites with the soul in its fullness. Grace is the soul and the spirit making love. Our higher self perceives grace embodied and enacted by others. Our soul notices grace as equanimity, balance, and beauty. Our soul recognizes grace as light, hope, and connection between the real and the unreal.

A number of years ago, a high fever alerted my doctors and me to a possible infection after I had laparoscopic abdominal surgery. My diaphragm was already not working well due to a side effect of the surgery. The fever raged. I struggled to breathe. Desperation for air triggered my fight-flight system into full alarm mode. Diagnosed with a bacterial infection in my blood, I felt so ill that I sensed I could die. I held on to my husband, Eric, hoping that his hand could carry me through and keep me alive.

My father, a retired pediatrician, came to see me. Here we were, three doctors, but I could not advocate for myself. As my condition continued to deteriorate, my father and Eric's concern developed into grief. My father, a devout Catholic, recommended that we recite the rosary. We agreed.

That night, surrendered to exhaustion and the possibility that I could die, I received my first dose of antibiotics. Shortly after, I fell asleep. While sleeping, something miraculous happened. A most powerful and loving presence held me and lifted my body. Gone was the heaviness. Gone was the struggle to breathe. My lungs stretched to the tips of my toes. Every breath I took filled not just the alveoli in my respiratory system but alveoli that expanded all over my body. There, raised up and breathing more freely, I was held in this space of love and healing. I felt a complete lightness of being, and I received grace.

I woke and immediately shared with Eric that I was going to be okay, that I felt embraced by grace, love, light, and hope. I had an exuberance of joy that I had never experienced, despite having had the amazing honor and overwhelming joy of giving birth to my children.

I could have interpreted this occurrence as a scientist and offered myself an analysis of how inflammation affected my brain to create this frequently described near death experience by ill and dying humans before me. Yet, I truly believed this was not a moment for science. There, in my room, a place for hope, healing, and love materialized. I was love and not afraid. That mystical sensation, that feeling of grace, was present when I awoke that day and remains with me to this day. Something in my consciousness shifted in me forever and affects how I live and interpret my life.

Gratitude

Each morning I feel gratitude and delight that I have one more day to savor my delicious morning latte. Cubans love good coffee. I am no exception. I appreciate that my dear husband makes great lattes every morning.

The dictionary defines gratitude as the quality of being thankful. Gratitude is the readiness to show appreciation and to return kindness to another. Gratitude allows us to focus on the good we are experiencing or receiving. Expressing gratitude allows us to define and deepen the meaning and significance of what we value and acknowledge, what brings us reward and joy.

When my girls were in elementary and middle school, I asked them at the end of their school year what they liked about their teachers and their classroom. I encouraged them to remember specific moments and qualities. Then I asked them to write a letter to thank and express their appreciation to give to their teachers on the last day of school. Taking the time to reflect on and express gratitude developed a deeper sense of awareness of their experiences and led to long lasting friendships with their teachers for years afterward. My daughters are skilled to function well in the world because of the dedicated work and contributions of their teachers and mentors. Teachers, like doctors, are interested in making a difference for learners. We need to express thanks for their work and the challenges and stresses they endure, which many of us became more aware of during and after the Covid-19 pandemic.

Research shows that the practice of gratitude can reduce depression and stress. When we decrease our perception of stress, we can turn off the fight-flight system. When we regulate our emotional system like this, we decrease our cortisol level. We also improve and increase our sense of calm and the quality of our sleep. Practicing gratitude improves our well-being.

When one of my daughters was a junior in high school, she attended a lecture by Tal Ben-Shahar, best-selling author of the book *Happier*. Inspired by the lecture, she began writing down three things that she was grateful for before bedtime. After three weeks of this practice, she noted feeling happier and less burdened by her heavy academic load. She now works as a physician-scientist. Recently, I asked her why she felt her ongoing gratitude practice still helps her. She explained that expressing gratitude enables her brain and neuronal pathways to shift focus and acknowledge all that is positive and good about her day, which counteracts the negative or tough occurrences in her day.

In fact, Dr. Rick Hanson, in his book *Hardwiring Happiness*, presents evidence that our ancestral brain has a predilection to focus more on what is bad and dangerous than what is good, in order to help us survive. Our brains are hardwired to have a negative bias, so it is upon us, with our conscious awareness, to counteract this negative outlook. If we look, we can find the kindness of humanity in the acts of others. We can change our attitude as to how we receive what life gives us. We can identify why our existence matters and helps others and ourselves. Changing our attitude and reflecting in this way empowers us to create meaning to enhance our lives.

This is beautifully demonstrated in Viktor Frankl's book, *Man's Search for Meaning*, which is about his survival as a prisoner in a Nazi concentration camp. His book describes how everyday life impacted the mind of prisoners. He asserts that the way prisoners imagined their future affected their longevity. We learn in this book that active positivity training—finding ways to make positive meaning out of even our most difficult experiences, is a way to declare that we are all born with a purpose, that our lives and the lives of those we interact with matter. Frankl's scientific theory, called logotherapy, is based on the premise that attempting to find meaning in our lives is one of the most powerful driving forces in humans. Meaning-making heals everyone, improves the quality of our lives, and cultivates a soulful existence.

As I reflect on my mother's journey through 15 years of Alzheimer's disease, I realize how her fortitude and equanimity in the midst of suffering, and her slow disconnection from us, expanded our awareness and developed us. I believe she hung on all those years because she felt her purpose in life was not done. Indeed, her presence made us all more accepting, curious, giving, forgiving, and compassionate people.

Gratitude is one of the most powerful practices to enhance our ability to create joy and make meaning about the value and significance of our life. Gratitude practices can be seen as trite. I want to give you a nuanced perspective. Consider just being happy about what you see, receive and experience. Just that. There are many easy ways to express and practice gratitude. We can journal about being grateful. We can express our thanks verbally. We can write letters to appreciate others and the difference their presence and actions make. We can send thank you notes or texts letting others know that we appreciate their efforts. We can meditate on the good aspects of our lives. We can send loving mettas—positive energy and kindness—to others with our minds. We can accept compliments and appreciation from others gracefully. We can create family or personal statements that remind us how blessed we are.

My Loving-Kindness Wish for You

May you feel spirit energy in your body
May your soul grow in infinite ways
May you allow yourself the time to reflect
May you feel dignity in your work
May you have a long health-span and soulful life

Meditation to Enhance Your Journaling

Please scan the QR Code with your Smartphone
or follow this link: https://youtu.be/DNaGi2sdrO8

Journaling for Transformation

Connecting to Spirit and Tending the Soul

- How do you define spirituality?
- In what ways are you spiritual?
- How do you define the soul?
- What is your life mythology?
- Think of one to three people in your life that you have loved or admired. What qualities did they display that made you feel their love? What about them that made you feel inspired?
- Have you ever had a time where the world stopped for you? How did you feel? Did you ever have a near end-of-life experience? If so, how were you changed by this, if at all?
- What are the things that give you joy and deepen the meaning of your life?
- Would you enjoy your work more if you believed that you and your work matter because it serves others? How can you engage more with your worthiness as a human and the value you offer with your presence in the world?
- Observe people and events. Be on the lookout for sightings of grace.
- Take the time to let a person know when you notice the generous qualities of their soul.
- What are your own soul qualities?
- How can you grow beyond your comfort zone?
- From reading the book and reflecting on Figure 7, what are your required components to have a soulful life?

Components of Vibrant Health

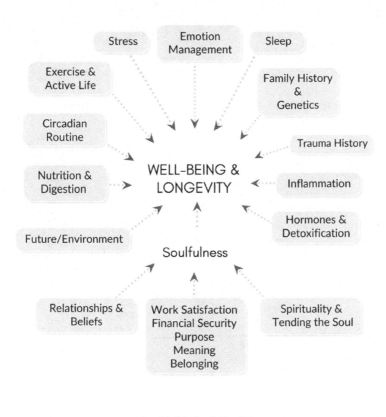

Stress

Emotion Management

Sleep

Exercise & Active Life

Family History & Genetics

Circadian Routine

Trauma History

Nutrition & Digestion

WELL-BEING & LONGEVITY

Inflammation

Future/Environment

Hormones & Detoxification

Soulfulness

Relationships & Beliefs

Work Satisfaction
Financial Security
Purpose
Meaning
Belonging

Spirituality & Tending the Soul

Figure 7. Components that affect our capacity to achieve a long healthy lifespan and a soulful life.

I hope our journey through the beautiful workings of our mind, body, and spirit helps you to become an advocate for yourself and your wellness and to see life in a more expansive way. I am deeply grateful that you have taken the time to be and learn with me. My deepest wish is that you continue to explore and implement the secrets I have shared with you so that you become creators of the most spectacular life—a life of wellness, connection, and purpose.

Acknowledgements

It took a village to help me evolve to this stage in my life. It took another village to write this book and offer you this simple Spiritual and Scientific Guide to Wellness. I have been blessed to be able to distill down to the essence what all of my teachers, mentors, coaches, family and friends, patients and collaborators have bestowed on me. I am an expression of the extensive insights, teachings, wisdom, love, and support of many individuals in my personal and professional life. Various challenges and difficulties have educated and caused me to seek out solutions, look higher and cultivate hope. These trials have enabled me to develop courage, grit, and resilience—all of which have helped me to overcome the grief, loss, and disappointments that are part of life.

I am profoundly grateful to Kim Douglas, founder of Write to Unite (www.write2unite.org), for taking on my manuscript. She encouraged me to reveal my more vulnerable stories as they connect us to each other and reveal to us our shared humanity. She advised me on how to restructure, revise and edit the book to make the information more accessible to a wider general audience. Kim's intuition, patience, love, and professionalism in giving birth to this book are admirable and lovingly magical. I thank Janice Nelson, Write to Unite's senior editor, for her loving support, expert scientific editing, fact checking, line-editing and especially her belief in this book, which she called the new *Red Tent*. I also appreciate Anisa Everett and Mitra Milani Engan who also brought their editorial expertise to the manuscript.

I thank Becky Norwood of Spotlight Publishing House for her expertise in the process of publishing the book. I thank her team, especially Maggie Mongan for creating the media platforms to give the book visibility so that millions of people may benefit from it.

I thank Barry Nalebuff for asking thoughtful questions and helping me realize that the book needed more suggestions from me as an expert in metabolism. I thank Catherine Lavoie and Eric J. Olson for reading and editing varied versions of the book.

Thanks to Matt Rudnitsky, Founder of Platypus Publishing, who challenged me to sit down every day for 3 months in order to finish writing the first draft of this 20-year-in-the-making book.

Appreciation and gratitude to the following individuals for their support:

Anne Ellis for superb support and expert editing of the first iteration of this book.

Philip Nicholas and Catherine Lavoie for their light in helping me in the creation of a related online course, Elevate Health and Wellness with Dr. Beatriz Olson at www.integrativebeing.org.

Joann Burnham, founder of Dharma Yoga in Nantucket for her light, her yoga and wise suggestions for the book.

My talented graphic designer and webmaster, Amanda Wolf, for creating our initial cover, all chapter figures and web design for the online-courses I teach.

Photographers Kris Kinsley Hancock at Nantucket Pix and Johnathon Henninger for the professional photographs for this book and other related media and courses.

My academic medicine teachers and supporters of my professional growth: Ethel Siris, Wishwa Kapoor, Michael Karpf, Alan Robinson, Joseph Verbalis, the late Janet Amico, Lynnette Nieman, George Chrousos, Bruce Nisula, and the late Thomas Amatruda, among others.

My Jungian guides Irene Gad and Jean Olson.

My spiritual, meditation and consciousness teachers Tara Brach, Craig Hamilton, Pema Chodron, Jon Kabat Zinn, the late David Simon, Deepak Chopra, Seth Suihō Segall, Bante Heneropola, and the holy Dali Lama.

Deepak Chopra and Andrew Weil for teaching the concept of mind body and integrative medicine, respectively, and Jeffrey Bland for introducing my mind to functional medicine.

My coaches at the Institute for Women's Centered Coaching, Facilitation and Leadership who helped me reclaim my feminine voice and supported my professional training for Transformational Leadership Certification.

My mentor and founder of the Institute for Women's Centered Coaching, Facilitation and Leadership, the brilliant Dr. Claire Zammit, who has inspired me to continue to evolve and bring the highest version of myself to help others.

My feminine power mastery, professional leadership, and mastermind sisters for supporting me as I expanded my professional direction to help greater audiences.

Mark Waldman, Mary Morrisey and John Assaraf, who offered programs that helped me grow beyond my limited mindsets and old beliefs.

My patients whose trust humbles and inspires me to work harder so I may serve you better.

Pattie Bosco, Denise Lefton, Joanne Palladino, Josephine Anzardi, Janet Goldberg, Kim Sands, Sharon Houle, Wendy Gallagher, Hannah Judy Gretz, Anne Ellis, Heather Stone, Kim Sands, Nan Levey, Barbara Schafer, Cynthia Ryan, Jill Baudry, Sharon Barna, Beverly Egan, and Karley Schaffer for your support and presence as I developed my first online educational programs.

My colleague Dr. Glenda Callender for being a superb endocrine surgeon for my patients, and for our online master classes on health, thyroid and other endocrine topics.

Brad Perkins and Dr. Eric Olson for video editing and media support.

My office team who has kept my medical healing ship, Integrative Endocrinology, floating for decades Sarah Bachelor, Francis Moresey, Rita Lombardi, Janet Siegal, Rose Esmiol, and Kathy Rice.

My dear friends Jean Olson, Manolita (Chiqui) Rodriguez, Meriamne Singer, Catherine Lavoie, Margi Sermer, Dr. Michelle Roberts, Kathleen Carrano, Terri Clark, Greta Olson and Philip Nicholas have been there to support me, listen, love, help and teach.

Ana Brito and Frances Rosa for taking care of Papi now, and of Abuela and Mami so lovingly till the end.

My parents Fernando and Belkis for their sacrifices, belief, expectations, and love. To my siblings who, like me, had their own immigrant journey and rose to thrive and live the American dream.

My daughters Loren and Lyra, for their courage to become who they are meant to be, and for teaching me what matters most.

And thank you to my Eric who is my true north, my kind, inspirational, brilliant, and beautiful husband, my classmate, professional colleague and orthopedic surgeon, best friend, father of our daughters, my pilot and guide, my editor and thought partner for this book and all projects, and the person that makes me laugh, dance, discover and enjoy our life.

Resources for Mind Body Secrets

Try my grounding meditations made for each chapter of this book. They are calming and create mind-body-spirit alignment. Duration 4-9 minutes.

Meditation 1 for Chapter 1 with Dr. Beatriz
https://youtu.be/PQoGAnv75zk

Meditation 2 for Chapter 2 with Dr. Beatriz
https://youtu.be/gkyEtt-8piU

Meditation 3 for Chapter 3 with Dr. Beatriz
https://youtu.be/JJvvKMSR7Os

Meditation 4 for Chapter 4 with Dr. Beatriz
https://youtu.be/Dpw_v0z0P4k

Meditation 5 for Chapter 5 & 6 with Dr. Beatriz
https://youtu.be/_SgD_PRe0iQ

Meditation 6 for Chapter 7 with Dr. Beatriz
https://youtu.be/dP3LtZmgAqU

Meditation 7 for Chapter 8 with Dr. Beatriz
https://youtu.be/SuLBWdAHyq8

Meditation 8 for Chapter 9 with Dr. Beatriz
https://youtu.be/DNaGi2sdrO8

Meditation to connect to your emotions and tend to your needs with Dr. Beatriz for chapters 2 or 3.
https://youtu.be/wZ4CefYgkG8

QR code for all meditations in paperback book publication.

Meditation apps you can purchase online that I've tried and liked.

My family and patients have improved their mood, sleep, and wellness using these apps.

Balanceapp.com
Headspace.com
Calm.com
Stressreset.co

Great meditation teachers whose books and CD's you can find online:

Craig Hamilton: www.evolvingwisdom.com
Tara Brach: www.tarabrach.com
Joe Dispenza: www.drjoedispenza
Jack Kornfield: www.jackkornfield
Sharon Salzberg: www.sharonsalzberg.com
Jon Kabat-Zinn: www.jonkabat-zinn.com

Gadgets that help track your health, sleep, vitals, and metabolic markers which you can buy online:

1. **Sleeptracker-AI** has good information on sleep. You can get an app and device for under your mattress. I use this app.
2. Other gadgets that help monitor sleep and activity at different budgets:

- Fitbit Charge: www.fitbit.com
- Garmin viviosmart 4: www.garmin.com
- Oura Ring: www.ouraring.com
- Dreem: www.dreem.com

3. FreeStyle Libre 14-day glucose sensor and receiver/monitor (insurance does not pay for this if you don't have diabetes but it's not so expensive). https://www.freestyle.abbott/us-en/products/freestyle-14-day.html

4. Keto sticks or Keto Sensors to figure out how many hours you need to fast.

Understanding how our brain deals with early experiences, trauma, and incomplete or lost attachments can help us to nurture ourselves compassionately, so we may create our authentic and fully embodied selves now.

The following books and movies are excellent resources to further this understanding.
(Chapters 1-3, 7, and 8)

1. Kalsched, Donald. *The Inner World of Trauma: Archetypal Defenses of the Personal Spirit* (Routledge, 1996).

2. van der Kolk, Bessel A. *The Body Keeps the Score: Brain, Mind and Body in the Healing of Trauma* (Viking 2014).

3. Schwartz, Richard C. and Sweezy, Martha. *Internal Family Systems Therapy: Second Edition* (The Guilford Press 2019).

4. Schwartz, Richard C. *No Bad Parts: Healing Trauma and Restoring Wholeness with the Internal Family Systems Model* (Sounds True 2021).

5. *What the Bleep!?: Down the Rabbit Hole.* [Movie]. Dirs. Arntz, W., Chasse, B., and Vincente, M. (20th Century Fox, 2006).

6. *The Secret.* [Movie]. Dir. Herriot, D. (The Secret 2006).

Stress reduction resources and techniques.

1. Kabat-Zinn, Jon. *Guided Mindfulness Meditation* [Compact Discs]. (Sounds True, 2005).
2. Kabat-Zinn, Jon. *Wherever You Go, There You Are: Mindfulness Meditation in Everyday Life.* (Hyperion, 1994).
3. Kornfield, Jack. *The Inner Art of Meditation* [Audio]. (Sounds True, 1993).
4. Benson, Herbert and Klipper, Miriam. *The Relaxation Response.* (William Morrow & Co., 1976).
5. Guendelman, S., Medeiros, S., and Rampers, H. (March 6, 2017) Mindfulness and emotion regulation: Insights from neurobiological, psychological, and clinical studies. *Frontiers in Psychology*, 8:220.
   https://doi.org/10.3389/fpsyg.2017.00220
6. Gunaratana, Bhante Henepola. *Mindfulness in Plain English.* (Wisdom Publishing, 2002).
7. Baron, Jill. *Don't Mess with Stress: A Simple Guide to Managing Stress, Optimizing Health and Making the World a Better Place.* (2020)
8. Tierney, Isabelle and Nicolas, Philip. StressReset [App]. Stress Reset.
   www.stressreset.co
9. The Science of Stress: What it does to your brain and body—and how to beat it. (2021, May). *Scientific American Special Collector's Edition,* 30:2s.

Places to learn and participate in Mindfulness Meditation.

- Tarabrach.com
  Free guided meditations and useful lectures on humanity, healing, mindfulness. She is, for me, one of the best.
- https://www.ummhealth.org/center-mindfulness
  They offer courses on mindfulness-based stress reduction (MBSR) here. This is a program created by Jon Kabat-

Zinn. I took this course in 1997 and I can say it changed my life for the better.

Developing heartfulness, self-care and self-compassion to heal past trauma and the resulting protective and limiting mindsets, perfectionism, setting boundaries, and resilience.
(Chapters 1-3, 8, and 9)

1. Gilbert, Paul. (Ed.) and Simos, Gregoris (Ed.) *Compassion Focused Therapy* (1st ed). (Routledge, 2022).
2. Gilbert, Paul. *Mindful Compassion*. (New Harbinger, 2014).
3. Brach, Tara. *Radical Acceptance*. (Random House, 2002)
4. Remen, Rachel Naomi. *Kitchen Table Wisdom* (10th ed). (Riverhead Books, 2006).
5. Brach, Tara. *Radical Compassion*. (Penguin Life, 2019).
6. Tawwab, Nedra Glover. *Set Boundaries, Find Peace: A Guide to Reclaiming Yourself* (Tarcher Perigee, 2021).
7. Salzberg, Sharon. *Loving Kindness: The Revolutionary Art of Happiness*. (Shambhala, 2003)
8. Canfield, Jack, Shimoff, Marci, et al. *Chicken Soup for the Woman's Soul: Stories to Open the Heart and Rekindle the Spirits of Women* (1st ed). (Health Communications, 1996)
9. Groden, Claire. (June 6, 2016). Why women are afraid of failure. *Elle* https://www.elle.com/life-love/a36828/why-women-are-afraid-of-failure/

Mind-Body-Spirit medicine, consciousness, mindfulness, connection, intimacy, spirituality, and the soul.
(Chapters 1-3, 7, 8, and 9)

1. Turner, Kelly. *Radical Remission: Surviving Cancer Against All Odds*. (HarperOne, 2015).
2. Myss, Caroline. *Anatomy of the Spirit: The Seven Stages of Power and Healing*. (Harmony, 1996).

3. Pert, Candace. *Molecules of Emotion: Why You Feel the Way You Feel.* (Simon & Schuster, 1999).

4. Chopra, Deepak and Tanzi, Rudolph. *Super Brain: Unleashing the Explosive Power of Your Mind to Maximize Health, Happiness, and Spiritual Well-Being.* (Harmony, 2013).

5. Kabat-Zinn, Jon. *Mindful Meditation: Cultivating the Wisdom of Your Body and Mind.* [Audio Cassette]. (Nightingale-Conant, 1995).

6. Kabat-Zinn, Jon. *Wherever You Go There You Are: Mindfulness Meditation in Everyday Life.* (Hyperion, 1995).

7. Kabat-Zinn, Jon. *Full Catastrophe Living: Using the Wisdom of Your Body and Mind to Face Stress, Pain, and Illness.* (Delta, 1990).

8. Moore, Thomas. *Care of the Soul: A Guide for Cultivating Depth and Sacredness in Everyday Life* (25th Anniversary ed). (Harper Perennial, 2016).

9. Moore, Thomas. *Soulmates: Honoring the Mystery of Love and Relationship.* (Harper Perennial, 2016).

10. Ford, Arielle. *The Soulmate Secret: Manifest the Love of Your Life with the Law of Attraction.* (HarperOne, 2011).

11. Kangwana, Kadzo. *Noble soul: A Guide to Spiritual Growth for Women.* (Blue Lapiss Books, 2022).

12. Sansone, Randy and Sansone, Lori. (Nov. 2010). Gratitude and wellbeing: The benefits of appreciation. *Psychiatry,* 7:11. 18-22.

13. Komase Y., Watanabe, K., Hori, D., et al. (2021) Effects of gratitude intervention on mental health and well-being among workers: A systematic review. *Journal of Occupational Health,* 63:1. e12290. https://doi.org/10.1002/1348-9585.12290

14. Pratt, Misty. (2022, February 17) The science of gratitude. *Mindful.* https://www.mindful.org/the-science-of-gratitude/

15. Stefan Salzmann, Frank Euteneuer, Jana Strahler, et al. (2018, February) Optimizing expectations and

distraction leads to lower cortisol levels after acute stress. *Psychoneuroendocrinology,* 88.144-152

16. The Dalai Lama, Salzberg, S., et al. Goleman, Daniel (Ed.). *Healing Emotions: Conversations with the Dalai Lama on Psychology, Meditation, and the Mind-Body Connection (Core Teachings of Dalai Lama).* (Shambhala, 2020).

17. Salzberg, Sharon. *Faith: Trusting Your Deepest Experience.* (Riverhead, 2003)

18. Balboni, Tracy A., et al. (2022, July 12). Spirituality in serious illness and health. *JAMA* 328:2. 184-197. https://doi.org/10.1001/jama.2022.11086

19. Siegel, Dan. *Intraconnected: MWe (Me + We) as the Integration of self, Identity, and Belonging.* (W.W. Norton and Company, 2022).

The microbiome and diet and mind-body health.
(Chapters 4, 6, and 7)

1. Anderson, Scott C. *The Psychobiotic Revolution: Mood, Food, and the New Science of the Gut-Brain Connection.* (National Geographic, 2019).

2. Kelly, J.R., et al. (2016, May). Brain-gut-microbiota axis: challenges for translation in psychiatry. *Annals of Epidemiology* 26:5. 366-72. https://doi.org10.1016/j.annepidem.2016.02.008 Epub 2016 Mar 8.

3. Dinan, T.G., et al. (2013, November 15). Psychobiotics: a novel class of psychotropics. *Biological Psychiatry* 74:10. 720-726 https://doi.org/10.1016/j.biopsych.2013.05.001

4. Pierce, J.M. and Alviña, K. (2019, October). The role of inflammation and the gut microbiome in depression and anxiety. *Journal of Neuroscience Research.* 97:10. 1223-1241. https://doi.org/10.1002/jnr.24476

5. Groeger, D., et al. (2023, January). Interactions between symptoms and psychological status in irritable bowel

syndrome: An exploratory study of the impact of a probiotic combination. *Neurogastroenterology and Motility* 35:1. e14477.
https://doi.org/10.1111/nmo.14477

6. Wang, H., et al. (2019, July). Bifidobacterium longum 1714™ Strain Modulates Brain Activity of Healthy Volunteers During Social Stress. *American Journal of Gastroenterology* 114:7. 1152-1162.
    https://doi.org/10.14309/ajg.0000000000000203

7. Han, H., Yi, B., Zhong, R., *et al.* (2021, July 20). From gut microbiota to host appetite: gut microbiota-derived metabolites as key regulators. *Microbiome* 9:1. 162.
    https://doi.org/10.1186/s40168-021-01093-y

8. Bredesen, Dale E. *The End of Alzheimer's: The First Program to Prevent and Reverse Cognitive Decline* (1ˢᵗ ed). (Avery 2017).

9. Perlmutter, David. *Grain Brain: The Surprising Truth About Wheat, Carbs, and Sugar—Your Brain's Silent Killer.* (Little, Brown Spark, 2018).

Microbiome and thyroid autoimmune diseases (Hashimoto's and Grave's) disease.
(Chapters 4-6)

1. Ruggeri, R.M., et al. (2021). Influence of dietary habits on oxidative stress markers in Hashimoto's Thyroiditis. *Thyroid* 31:1. 96-105.
    https://doi.org/10.1089/thy.2020.0299

2. Zhao, F., Feng, J., and et al. (2018, February) Alterations of the gut microbiota in Hashimoto's thyroiditis patients. *Thyroid* 28:2. 175-186.
    https://doi.org/10.1089/thy.2017.0395

3. Jiang, W., Yu, X., et al. (2021, May) Gut microbiota may play a significant role in the pathogenesis of Graves' disease. *Thyroid* 31:5 810-820.
    https://doi.org/10.1089/thy.2020.0193

4. Dosiou, Chrysoula. (2020, April). Thyroid and Fertility: Recount advances. *Thyroid* 30:4. 479-486. https://doi.org/10.1089/thy.2019.0382

5. Dhillon-Smith, R.K., et al. (2020, August 1) The prevalence of thyroid dysfunction and autoimmunity in women with a history of miscarriage and subfertility. *Journal of Clinical Endocrinology and Metabolism* 105:8. 2667-2677. https://doi.org/10.1210/clinem/dgaa302

Prevention and lifesaving practices: diet, lifestyle, sleep, exercise, stress, and body-mind outcomes.
(Chapters 3-7)

1. Perlmutter, David. *Grain Brain: The Surprising Truth About Wheat, Carbs, and Sugar—Your Brain's Silent Killer.* (Little, Brown Spark, 2018).

2. Agus, David. *The End of Illness.* (Free Press, 2012).

3. Campbell, Collin and Campbell II, Thomas. *The China Study.* (Benbella, 2016).

4. Weil, Andrew. *Eight weeks to Optimum Health.* (Knopf, 1997).

5. Weil, Andrew. *Healthy Aging: A Lifelong Guide to Your Physical and Spiritual Well-Being.* (Knopf, 2005).

6. Blackburn, Elizabeth and Epel, Elissa. *The Telomere Effect: A Revolutionary Approach to Living Younger, Healthier, and Longer.* (Grand Central Publishing, 2017).

7. Amiri, Sohrab, et al. (2021, August). Effect of exercise training on improving sleep disturbances: a systematic review and meta-analysis of randomized control trials. *Sleep Medicine* 84. 205-218. https://doi.org/10.1016/j.sleep.2021.05.013

8. Reid, Kathryn J., et al. (2010, October). Aerobic exercise improves self-reported sleep and quality of life in older adults with insomnia. *Sleep Medicine* 11:9. 934-940.

9. Dolezal, Brett A., et al. (2017). Interrelationship between sleep and exercise: A systematic review. *Advances in Preventive Medicine* 2017:1364387.

https://doi.org/10.1155/2017/1364387

10. Woods, J.A., Wilund, K.R., et al. (2012,February). Exercise, inflammation and aging. *Aging and Disease* 3:1. 130–140.

11. Willett, W.C. and Ludwig, D.S. (2020, February, 13). Milk and Health. *New England Journal of Medicine* 382:7. 644-654.

12. Zheng, Guohua, et al. (2019, April 26). Effect of Aerobic Exercise on Inflammatory Markers in Health Middle-Aged and Older Adults: A Systematic Review and Meta-Analysis of Randomized Controlled Trials. *Frontiers in Aging and Neuroscience* 11 (*Sec. Neuroinflammation and Neuropath*). https://doi.org/10.3389/fnagi.2019.00098

Relationships, assumptions, negotiations, and dreams.
(Chapter 5, 8 and 9)

1. Luis, Don Miguel. *The Four Agreements: A Practical Guide to Personal Freedom (A Toltec Wisdom Book)*. (Amber-Allen, 1997). Impeccable speech. Don't take things personally. Don't make assumptions. Always do your best.

2. Jung, Carl G., Adler, Gerhard (Ed.). *Dreams*. (R. Hull, Trans). (Princeton University Press, 1974). ISBN 0-691-01792-1

3. Cooper J.C. *An Illustrated Encyclopedia of Traditional Symbols*. (Thames and Hudson, 1978).

4. Stoddard, Alexandra. *Living Beautifully Together*. (Harper Perennial, 1991).

5. Groden, Claire. (June 6, 2016). Why women are afraid of failure. *Elle*
https://www.elle.com/life-love/a36828/why-women-are-afraid-of-failure/

Positive Psychology, gratitude, purpose and meaning, and happiness can reframe your view of life.
(Chapters 8 and 9)

1. Ben-Shahar, Tal. *Happier: Learn the Secrets to Daily Joy and Lasting Fulfillment.* (McGraw Hill, 2007)
2. Seligman, Martin, et al. *Authentic Happiness: Using the New Positive Psychology to Realize Your Potential for Lasting Fulfillment.* (Free Press, 2002).
3. Positivepsychology.com
4. Salzberg, Sharon. *Real Happiness, 10ᵗʰ Anniversary Addition: A 28-Day Program to Realize the Power of Meditation.* (Workman Publishing, 2019).
5. Hanson, Rick. *Hardwiring Happiness: The New Brain Science of Contentment, Calm, and Confidence.* (Harmony, 2013). Re: Counteracting our ancestral brain's negativity bias.
6. Frankl, Viktor. *Man's Search for Meaning.* (Harmony, 2016).
7. Shimoff, Marci. *Happy for No Reason: 7 Steps to Being Happy from the Inside Out.* (Atria, 2009).

Diets: Nutrition, various diets, disease reversal or prevention, and resources
Chapters 5, 6 and 7.

1. www.DietDoctor.com
2. masteringdiabetes.com Plant-based program to reverse or prevent diabetes.
3. Esselstyn Jr, C., Sanders, F., et al. *Prevent and Reverse Heart Disease: The Revolutionary, Scientifically Proven, Nutrition-Based Cure.* (Avery, 2007).
4. Stone, Gene (Ed.). *Forks over Knives: The Plant-Based Way to Health.* (The Experiment, 2011).
5. Campbell, Collin and Campbell II, Thomas. *The China Study.* (Benbella, 2016).

6. Greger, Michael and Stone, Gene. *How Not to Die: Discover the Foods Scientifically Proven to Prevent and Reverse Disease.* (Flatiron Books, 2015).

7. Willett, W.C. and Ludwig, D.S. (2020, February, 13). Milk and Health. *New England Journal of Medicine* 382:7. 644-654.

8. Olson, Beatriz. (2016, August 11). Best type of high protein diet depends on your health. [Blog Post] https://beatrizolson.com/best-type-of-high-protein-diet-depends-on-your-health/

9. Bredesen, Dale E. *The End of Alzheimer's: The First Program to Prevent and Reverse Cognitive Decline* (1ˢᵗ ed). (Avery 2017).

10. Cabeca, Anna. *Keto-Green 16: The Fat-Burning Power of Ketogenic Eating + the Nourishing Strength of Alkaline Foods = Rapid Weight Loss and Hormone Balance.* (Ballantine, 2020)

11. Sisson, M., Kearns, B., et al. *The Keto-Reset Diet: Reboot Your Metabolism in 21 Days and Burn Fat Forever.* (Harmony, 2017).

12. Axe, Josh. *Keto Diet: Your 30-Day Plan to Lose Weight, Balance Hormones, Boost Brain Health, and Reverse Disease.* (Little, Brown Spark, 2019).

13. Masley, Steven. *The Mediterranean Method: Your Complete Plan to Harness the Power of the Healthiest Diet on the Planet—Lose Weight, Prevent Heart Disease, and More! (A Mediterranean Diet Cookbook).* (Harmony, 2019).

14. Cordain, Loren, *The Real Paleo Diet Cookbook: 250 All-New Recipes from the Paleo Expert.* (Harvest, 2015).

15. Willett, W.C. and Ludwig, D.S. (2020, February, 13). Milk and Health. *New England Journal of Medicine* 382:7. 644-654. https://doi.org/10.1056/NEJMra1903547

16. Średnicka-Tober, D., Barański, M., et al. (2016, March 28). Composition differences between organic and conventional meat: a systematic literature review and meta-analysis. *British Journal of Nutrition* 115:6. 994–1011. https://doi.org/10.1017/s0007114515005073

17. Hyman, Mark. *The Pegan Diet* (this is the most aligned to what I am promoting in this book with using whole foods and plant-dominant diet)

Weight gain, insulin excess and resistance, inflammation, inflammaging, oxidative stress, diabetes, aging, and interval fasting and other treatments to counteract the chaos of metabolic dissonance and diabetes reversal and prevention. (Chapters 4, 5, and 6)

1. Longo, Valter. *The Longevity Diet: Discover the New Science Behind Stem Cell Activation and Regeneration to Slow Aging, Fight Disease, and Optimize Weight.* (Avery, 2018).
2. ProLon through L-Nutra offers a 5-day fast-mimicking program (meal replacements for 1-5 days that fool the body into thinking that it is fasting) in two ways: one is anti-aging and cancer prevention www.prolonfmd.com and the second is about diabetes reversal L-Nutrahealth.com. Both work, though for diabetes reversal you must do a 5-day fast mimicking program every month and eat whole, healthy foods in between as I describe in this book. As an endocrinologist I use the latter as an option to weight loss meds and my patients get discounts on both programs. I am offering you this discount as well, click the link **http://www.prolonfmd.com/DrBeatrizOlson**, the discount will be reflected in the cart.
3. Fung, Jason. *The Obesity Code-Unlocking the Secrets of Weight Loss* (Book 1). (Greystone Books, 2016).
4. Fung, Jason. *The Diabetes Code: Prevent and Reverse Type 2 Diabetes Naturally (The Wellness Code, Book Two).* (Greystone, 2018).
5. Fung, Jason. *The Cancer Code: A Revolutionary New Understanding of a Medical Mystery (The Wellness Code, 3).* (Harper Wave, 2020).

6. Fung, Jason and Moore, Jimmy. *Complete Guide to Fasting: Heal Your Body Through Intermittent, Alternate-Day, and Extended Fasting.* (Victory Belt, 2016).
7. Sulaj, A., et al. (2022. August). Six-month periodic fasting in patients with type 2 diabetes and diabetic nephropathy: A proof-of-concept study. *The Journal of Clinical Endocrinology & Metabolism* 2022 107:8. 2167-2181. https://doi.org/10.1210/clinem/dgac197 Study used fast-mimicking program L-Nutra once a week for 6 months in diabetics with complications. Shows that fasting cycles can improve kidney disfunction in diabetics.
8. Tara, Sylvia. *The Secret Life of Fat: Science Behind the Body's Least Understood Organ and What It Means for You.* (W.W. Norton & Company, 2016).
9. De Cabo, M. and Mattson, MP. (2019, December 26). Effects of intermittent fasting on health, aging, and disease. *New England Journal of Medicine* 381. 2541-2551. https://doi.org/10.1056/nejmra1905136
10. Mercola, Joseph. *Effortless Healing: 9 Simple Ways to Sidestep Illness, Shed Excess Weight, and Help Your Body Fix Itself.* (Harmony, 2015).
11. Yang, X., Zhou, J., Shao, H., et al. (2022, December 14). Effect of an intermittent calorie-restricted diet on type 2 diabetes remission: A randomized controlled trial. *The Journal of Clinical Endocrinology & Metabolism* dgac661. https://doi.org/10.1210/clinem/dgac661
12. Gentileschi, P. et al. (2021). Metabolic surgery for type II diabetes: an update. *Acta Diabetologica* 58. 1153-9.
13. Shmerling, R. ((2020, May 26). When dieting doesn't work. [Blog]. https://www.health.harvard.edu/blog/when-dieting-doesnt-work-2020052519889
14. Ge, L., Sadeghirad, B., et al. (2020, April 1). Comparison of dietary macronutrient patterns of 14 popular named dietary programmes for weight and cardiovascular risk factor reduction in adults: systematic review and network

meta-analysis of randomised trials. *British Medical Journal* 369:m696.
https://doi.org/10.1136/bmj.m696

15. Hazzard VM, Telke SE, Simone M, Anderson LM, Larson NI, Neumark-Sztainer D. Intuitive eating longitudinally predicts better psychological health and lower use of disordered eating behaviors: findings from EAT 2010-2018. Eat Weight Disord. 2021 Feb;26(1):287-294. doi: 10.1007/s40519-020-00852-4

16. Sandra Aamodt: *Why Dieting Doesn't Usually Work.* [Video]. (TED Talk).

17. Freedhoff, Y. and Hall, K.D. (2016, August 27). Weight loss diet studies: we need help not hype. *Lancet* 388:10047. 849-851.
https://doi.org/10.1016/S0140-6736(16)31338-1

18. Mozaffarian, D., Hao, T., et al. (2011, June 23). Changes in diet and lifestyle and long-term weight gain in women and men. New England Journal of Medicine 364. 2392-2404
https://doi.org/10.1056/NEJMoa1014296

19. Li, X., Perelman, D., et al. (2022, December 20). Distinct factors associated with short-term and long-term weight loss induced by low-fat or low-carbohydrate diet intervention. *Cell Reports Medicine* 3:12. 100870.
https://doi.org/10.1016/j.xcrm.2022.100870

20. Sinclair, David. *Lifespan: Why We Age—and Why We Don't Have To.* (Atria, 2019).

21. Diaz-Vegas, A., et al. (2020, June 3). Is mitochondrial dysfunction a common root of noncommunicable chronic diseases? *Endocrine Reviews* 41:3. bnaa005.
https://doi.org/10.1210/endrev/bnaa005

22. Kowaltowski, A.J., and Vercesi, A.E. (1999, February 26). Mitochondrial damage induced by conditions of oxidative stress. *Free Radical Biology and Medicine* 26:3-4. 463-471.
https://doi.org/10.1016/s0891-5849(98)00216-0

23. Miwa, S., et.al. (2022, July 1). Mitochondrial dysfunction in cell senescence and aging. *Journal of Clinical Investigation* 132:13. e158447. https://doi.org/10.1172/JCI158447.

Obesity and (adipose tissue) Fat Cells

1. *Adult obesity facts.* (Accessed 2022, July 26). Centers for Disease Control and Prevention. https://www.cdc.gov/obesity/data/adult.html

2. Ward, Z.J., Bleich, S.N., Cradock, A.L., et al. (2019, December 19). Projected US state-level prevalence of adult obesity and severe obesity. *New England Journal of Medicine* *381*:25. 2440-2450. https://doi:10.1056/NEJMsa1909301

3. Weir, C.B. and Jan, A. [Internet]. BMI classification percentile and cut off points. (StatPearls, Accessed 2022, May 17 updated 2022, June 27). https://www.ncbi.nlm.nih.gov/books/NBK541070

4. Hales, C.M., Fryar, C.D., et al. (2018, April 24). Trends in obesity and severe obesity prevalence in US youth and adults by sex and age, 2007-2008 to 2015-2016. *JAMA* 319:16 1723-1725. https://doi.org/10.1001/jama.2018.3060

5. Christakis, N.A. and Fowler, J.H. (2007, July 26). The spread of obesity in a large social network over 32 years. *New England Journal of Medicine* 357. 370-9. https://doi.org/10.1056/NEJMsa066082

6. Cypess, A.M. (2022, February 24). Reassessing Human Adipose Tissue. *New England Journal of Medicine* 386:8. 768-779. https://doi.org/10.1056/NEJMra2032804

7. Creanga, A.A., et al. (2022, July 21). Obesity in pregnancy. *New England Journal of Medicine* 387:3. 248-259. https://doi.org/10.1056/NEJMra1801040

8. Halberg, N., et al. (2008, September). The adipocyte as an endocrine cell. *Endocrinology and Metabolism Clinics of North America* 37:3. 753-68. https://doi.org/10.1016/j.ecl.2008.07.002

9. Good discussion on weight bias and outcomes. Be fit with intuitive eating. Urtha, Jules (2022, January, 31). Asking your patients to lose weight may do more harm than good. Here's why. [Internet]. https://www.mdlinx.com/article/asking-your-patients-to-lose-weight-may-do-more-harm-than-good-heres-why/5DvQsSAofZJXdC2Jo7o47O

10. Pearl, R.L. and Schulte, E.M. (2021, June). Weight bias during the covid-19 pandemic. *Current Obesity Reports* 10:2. 181-190. https://doi.org/10.1007/s13679-021-00432-2

11. Lawrence, B.J., Kerr, D., et al. (2021). Weight bias among health care professionals: A systematic review and meta-analysis. *Obesity* 29:11. 1802-1812. https://doi.org/10.1002/oby.23266

12. Jastreboff, A.M., et al. (2022, July 21). Tirzepatide once weekly for the treatment of Obesity. *New England Journal of Medicine* 387:3. 205-216. https://doi.org/10.1056/NEJMoa2206038

13. Hall, K.D., Kahan, S. (2018, January). Maintenance of lost weight and long-term management of obesity. Medical Clinics of North America 102:1. 183-197. https://doi.org/10.1016/j.mcna.2017.08.012

Factors affecting aging: telomeres, lifespan, and mortality and how to deal with it all to improve the quality of our lives and aging. (Chapters 4-9)

1. Atul Gawande. *Being Mortal: Medicine and What Matters in the End.* (Metropolitan Books, 2014).

2. Chopra, Deepak and Tanzi, Rudolph. *Super Brain: Unleashing the Explosive Power of Your Mind to Maximize*

Health, Happiness, and Spiritual Well-Being. (Harmony, 2013).

3. Sinclair, David. *Lifespan: Why We Age—and Why We Don't Have To.* (Atria, 2019).

4. Blackburn, Elizabeth and Epel, Elissa. *The Telomere Effect: A Revolutionary Approach to Living Younger, Healthier, and Longer.* (Grand Central Publishing, 2017).

5. Bredesen, Dale E. *The End of Alzheimer's: The First Program to Prevent and Reverse Cognitive Decline* (1st ed). (Avery 2017).

6. Turner, Kelly. *Radical Remission: Surviving Cancer Against All Odds.* (HarperOne, 2015).

7. www.Deepakchopra.com

8. Athanasoulia-Kaspar, A.P., et al. (2018, August 1). Shorter telomeres associated with high doses of glucocorticoids: the link to increased mortality? *Endocrine Connections* 7:11. 1217–1226.
https://doi.org/10.1530/EC-18-0362

9. Lee, Duk-Chul and Im, Jee-Aee, et al. (2005, August 31). Effect of long-term hormone therapy on telomere length of postmenopausal women. *Yonsei Medical Journal* 46:4. 471–479.
https://doi.org/10.3349/ymj.2005.46.4.471

10. Shin, Yun-A and Lee, Kyoung-Young. (2016, June, 30). Low estrogen levels and obesity are associated with shorter telomere lengths in pre- and postmenopausal women. *Journal of Exercise Rehabilitation* 12:3. 238-246.
https://doi.org/10.12965/jer.1632584.292

11. Cheung, A.S., Yeap, B.B., et al. (2017, October). Effects of androgen deprivation therapy on telomere length. *Clinical Endocrinology* 87:4. 381-385. [published online 2017, May 24].
https://doi.org/10.1111/cen.13382

12. Fadnes, L.T., Økland, J-M, et al. (2022, February, 8). Estimating impact of food choices on life expectancy: A modeling study. *PLoS Medicine* 19:2. e1003889.

https://doi.org/10.1371/journal.pmed.1003889
13. Asprey, Dave. *Smarter Not Harder: The Biohacker's Guide to Getting the Body and Mind You Want*
14. Hyman, Mark. *Young for Ever*

Resting energy expenditure and metabolic rate adaptations as we lose hormones, age, or get stressed.
(Chapters 3-7)

1. Day, D.S., et al. (2005, June 1). Sex hormone suppression reduces resting energy expenditure and β-Adrenergic support of resting energy expenditure *The Journal of Clinical Endocrinology & Metabolism* 90:6. 3312–3317. https://doi.org/10.1210/jc.2004-1344
   GNRH suppresses axis in normal menstruant women, and this is what happens (1405 ± 42 *vs.* 1376 ± 43 kcal/d; 5878 ± 176 *vs.* 5757 ± 180 kJ/d; $P = 0.05$). There were no differences in respiratory exchange ratio (RER).
2. Melanson, E.L., et al. (2015, November 1). Regulation of energy expenditure by estradiol in premenopausal women. *Journal of Applied Physiology* 119:9. 975-81. https://doi.org/10.1152/japplphysiol.00473.2015
   (Total energy expenditure -128 cals/day GNRH AG and estrogen therapy replacement can prevent this slowing of resting energy metabolism).
3. Jones, A., et al. (2004, May 1). Body-composition differences between African American and white women: relation to resting energy requirements. *The American Journal of Clinical Nutrition* 79:5. 780–786. https://doi.org/10.1093/ajcn/79.5.780
4. Alfonzo-González, G., Doucet, E., et al. (2006, January). Greater than predicted decrease in resting energy expenditure with age: cross-sectional and longitudinal evidence. *European Journal of Clinical Nutrition* 60:1. 18–24. https://doi.org/10.1038/sj.ejcn.1602262

5. Kiecolt-Glaser, J.K, et al. (2015, April 1). Daily stressors, past depression, and metabolic responses to high-fat meals: A novel path to obesity. *Biological Psychiatry* 77:7. 653-660. https://doi.org/10.1016/j.biopsych.2014.05.018 (stress and decrease of energy expenditure of 100 cals/day).

6. Nayor, M., Chernofsky, A., et al. (2021, November 21). Physical activity and fitness in the community: the Framingham Heart Study. *European Heart Journal* 42:4. 4565–4575. https://doi.org/10.1093/eurheartj/ehab580 [Published: August 26, 2021]

7. Shea, K.L., Gavin, K.M., et al. (2015, October). Body composition and bone mineral density after ovarian hormone suppression with or without estradiol treatment. *Menopause* 22:10. 1045 1052. https://doi.org/10.1097/GME.0000000000000430 (bone loss + Increased visceral fat mass)

For women and the men who care: Hormone replacement and women empowerment topics. How to thrive and mature beautifully with a long and healthy lifespan.
(Chapter 1-3, 6, and 7)

1. Beatriz Olson discusses *Menopause Transition* [Video]. https://youtu.be/XD0JnGARXpI
2. Beatriz Olson discusses *Testosterone Replacement* [Video]. https://youtu.be/tmE9Y7e0mHA
3. Beatriz Olson discusses why there is no testosterone available for women, other than men's preparations, in 2023. [Blog]. https://beatrizolson.com/why-is-there-no-fda-approved-testosterone-for-women-news-about-my-own-published-research-on-testosterone-for-women/
4. Beatriz Olson discusses bioidentical hormones. *What Are They? Should You Have Them Replaced?* [Video]. https://youtu.be/vo1RZ5mUq9Q

5. Nagoski, Emily. *Come as you Are: The Surprising New Science that Will Transform Your Sex Life.* (Simon & Schuster, 2015).

6. Ross, Sherry A. *She-ology: The Definitive Guide to Women's Intimate Health. Period.* (Savio Republic, 2017).

7. Northrup, Christiane. *Women's Bodies, Women's Wisdom: Creating Physical and Emotional Health and Healing.* (Bantam, 2020).

8. Berman, J., Bumiller, E., and Berman, L. *For Women Only, Revised Edition: A Revolutionary Guide to Reclaiming Your Sex Life.* (Holt Paperbacks, 2005).

9. Cabeca, Anna. *The Hormone Fix: Burn Fat Naturally, Boost Energy, Sleep Better, and Stop Hot Flashes, the Keto-Green Way.* (Ballantine, 2019).

10. Gottfried, Sara. *The Hormone Cure: Reclaim Balance, Sleep and Sex Drive; Lose Weight; Feel Focused, Vital, and Energized Naturally with the Gottfried Protocol.* (Scribner, 2013).

11. https://beatrizolson.com/ [Website]. Blogs on HRT, testosterone, hypothyroid, Hashimoto's, Grave's disease, weight, and much more.

12. Vliet, Elizabeth Lee. *The Savvy Woman's Guide to Testosterone: How to Revitalize Your Sexuality, Strength and Stamina.* (HER Place, 2005).

13. Mok, Charles. *Testosterone: Strong Enough for A Man, Made for A Woman.* (ForbesBooks, 2017).

14. Comite, Florence. *Keep it up: The Power of Precision Medicine to Conquer Low T and Revitalize Your Life!* (Rodale, 2013). For men and the women who love them.

15. Moore, Donnica and Jarvis, Sarah (Ed.). *Women's Health for Life.* (Dorling Kindersley 2009). I am a contributing author in this book! (You can find me in chapter 3 - Staying Well and Chapter 14 - Endocrinology and Metabolism).

Other Possibilities to Grow

You can connect with Dr. Beatriz by taking her course. Click the link to learn more. www.integrativebeing.org

If you would like to have a consultation with Dr. Beatriz, please click this link which will take you to her website www.beatrizolson.com

About the Author

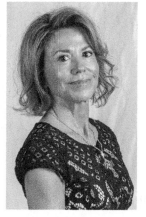

Dr. Beatriz Olson is a superbly trained endocrinologist who also has unique and extraordinary skills in mind body medicine and transformative health empowerment.

Her training as an academic clinician focuses on holistic healing, experience running an integrative medicine community in Connecticut for 15 years, and 3-decades of experience and expertise caring for patients set her apart from others.

Her approach to healthcare combines evidence-based science, mind-body-spirit aligning techniques, and integrative and functional medicine to provide comprehensive and effective healing. With expertise and compassion informed by being a Cuban immigrant, Dr. Olson has transformed the health and well-being of thousands of patients.

Dr. Olson is board-certified in Endocrinology, Metabolism & Diabetes and Internal Medicine, and has certifications in Age Management Medicine and Feminine Power Transformational Leadership.

Dr. Olson graduated from Barnard College, Columbia University College of Physicians and Surgeons, and did her residency in internal medicine and research-clinical fellowship in Endocrinology at the University of Pittsburgh. She served as clinician-scientist at the National Institutes of Health and later as teaching-faculty at Yale University School of Medicine. Dr. Olson has numerous first-authored publications in basic science and clinical peer-reviewed journals and contributed chapters to several textbooks. *Mind Body Secrets: A Medical Doctor's Spiritual and Scientific Guide to Wellness* is the first integrative medicine book she has written for a general audience. Dr. Olson resides in Connecticut with her husband, Dr. Eric J. Olson.

Embrace the New You

and

Celebrate Your New

Empowered and Healthy Life!

Made in the USA
Las Vegas, NV
01 March 2024

86460832R00148